THE NATURAL WAY SERIES

Increasing numbers of people worldwide are falling victim to illnesses which modern medicine, for all its technical advances, seems often powerless to prevent – and sometimes actually causes. To help with these so-called 'diseases of civilization' more and more people are turning to 'natural' medicine for an answer. The *Natural Way* series aims to offer clear, practical and reliable guidance to the safest, gentlest and most effective treatments available – and so to give sufferers and their families the information they need to make their own choices about the most suitable treatments.

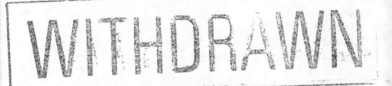

Titles in The Natural Way *series*

Allergies
Arthritis & Rheumatism
Asthma
Back Pain
Cancer
Candida
Chronic Fatigue Syndrome
Colds & Flu
Cystitis
Diabetes
Eczema
Epilepsy
Hay Fever
Heart Disease
HIV & AIDS
Irritable Bowel Syndrome
Infertility
Migraine
Multiple Sclerosis
Premenstrual Syndrome
Psoriasis

THE NATURAL WAY

Candida

Simon Martin

Series medical consultants
Dr Peter Albright MD (USA)
& Dr David Peters MD (UK)

Approved by the
AMERICAN HOLISTIC MEDICAL ASSOCIATION
& BRITISH HOLISTIC MEDICAL ASSOCIATION

ELEMENT

Shaftesbury, Dorset • Boston, Massachusetts
Melbourne, Victoria

© Element Books Limited 1998
Text © Simon Martin 1998

First published in the UK in 1998 by
Element Books Limited
Shaftesbury, Dorset SP7 8BP

Published in the USA in 1998 by
Element Books, Inc.
160 North Washington Street,
Boston, MA 0211

Published in Australia in 1998 by
Element Books and distributed by
Penguin Australia Limited
487 Maroondah Highway,
Ringwood, Victoria 3134

Reprinted 1999 (twice)

Cover Design by Slatter-Anderson
Text illustrations by David Woodroffe
Designed by Roger Lightfoot
Typeset by Intype London Ltd
Printed and bound in Great Britain by
Caledonian International Book Manufacturing

British Library Cataloguing in Publication
data available

Library of Congress Cataloging in Publication Data available

ISBN 1 86204 193 8

Contents

List of Illustrations

To naturopaths Leon Chaitow and John Stirling with thanks for their continuing inspiration and dedication.

Acknowledgements

Many thanks to Leon Chaitow, ND, for taking the lid off the candida story in the UK. I echo his appreciation of the candida pioneers Dr C. Orian Truss, MD, and Dr William G. Crook, MD and add my own for the work of John Stirling, Jane McWhirter and Gill Jacobs in the UK. I'd also like to thank Richard Thomas for the initial idea, Grace Cheetham of Element for much help in turning it into words on paper, series consultants Dr David Peters and Dr Peter Albright for their valuable suggestions, and Dr Peter J. D'Adamo for my high-energy diet.

Introduction

Candida is a naturally occurring yeast that only becomes
a problem when it gets out of control. There are more
than 80 strains of candida, of which *Candida albicans* is
the most common. Most people know of it as thrush, a
yeast infection of the genitals; in fact it is a normal inhabi-
tant of the mouth, intestinal tract, skin and vagina.

Candida's numbers are normally kept in balance – and
the yeast kept in its place – by a mass of 'friendly'
bacteria that live inside us and stop it from overpopula-
ting us. Our immune systems, of which these 'friendly'
bacteria are technically a part, also keep it in check. But
under certain circumstances, typically after a course of
antibiotics and helped by a diet high in sugar, it grows
and spreads.

Here we run into the first problem with candida.
Doctors disagree about the extent to which it can spread.
The conventional view is that it commonly involves the
vagina, the skin, the mouth or the respiratory tract, and
that it is extremely rare for it to spread throughout the
body. It is known that it can spread, but many pro-
fessionals associate this systemic overgrowth with
extreme situations such as AIDS, where it has been estimated that 80 per cent of patients have severe infection
with candida, or in cancer patients receiving chemotherapy. In these sort of situations, it can have fatal
consequences.

In contrast, other doctors and researchers believe that
systemic candida overgrowth is much more common
than is generally realized. It is not fatal and certainly

nowhere near as serious as AIDS, but it does signify that a sufferer's immune system is not up to scratch and warrants being taken more seriously than thrush. This is the view of many natural health practitioners, particularly nutritional therapists and naturopaths, who regularly treat patients for this type of candida overgrowth.

These practitioners believe the research shows that candida is a dynamic, opportunistic parasite that, like many other micro-organisms which have evolved strategies to survive in and on the human body, is often able to outwit attempts by our in-built defence mechanisms to dislodge it. Even the 'friendly' bacteria in our gut may be unable to re-establish the balance of power that keeps candida from spreading.

This view takes account of the fact that candida has a fungal form, enabling it to put down root-like structures into the wall of the intestines. When this happens, it can allow partly digested food particles, as well as waste products and naturally occurring toxins, into the bloodstream, where they provoke physiological reactions and affect the immune system. Many practitioners believe that this is a major cause of food allergies and intolerances.

This is not the low-key, localized infection that most people are familiar with, but an overgrowth that it is claimed can have dramatic and far-reaching effects on health. These problems are not confined to the digestive tract, where candida can cause bloating and indigestion, but can show up anywhere in the body, causing muscle pain, breathing problems or migraines, for instance, or even affect the mind, mood and emotions and cause depression, inability to concentrate or memory loss. There may be allergy-type reactions such as catarrh, sneezing and symptoms similar to hay fever as well as conditions such as chronic fatigue and pain.

Yeast treatment expert Dr William Crook, the former visiting professor at Ohio State and other universities,

and author of the classic 1983 book *The Yeast Connection*
lays the blame for candida firmly at the door of antibiotics. He has continued to research the condition and
its treatment since his first meetings with Dr C. Orian
Truss in 1979. He says:

> Many different factors play a part in making you sick, yet
> I am convinced that repeated courses of broad-spectrum
> antibiotics are the main 'villain'. These antibiotics cause yeast
> overgrowth in your intestinal tract and vaginal yeast infec-
> tions. And these infections, like a stream cascading down a
> mountain, set off disturbances which can make you feel 'sick
> all over'.

In Dr Crook's picture of candida overgrowth there is
little mystery, just a logical sequence of effects, leading
from one to the next: from antibiotics to a wipe-out of
helper bacteria, to Candida overgrowth producing toxins
which weaken the immune system which means you
may get an infection, which leads to antibiotics . . . and
on round the vicious cycle. Or to give Dr Crook's complete scenario, from antibiotics to candida overgrowth to:

- weakened immune system
- nutritional deficiencies
- food allergies
- digestive disturbances and involvement of the
  nervous system, endocrine system (your glands) and
  respiratory system, and activation of viruses and parasites that had been held in check by a well-nourished
  body . . .

A mass of apparently unrelated symptoms follow,
including

- headache
- depression
- low body temperature
- infertility
- sexual dysfunction
- pre-menstrual problems

- more nutritional disturbances,
- chronic fatigue
- poor memory
- anxiety
- sleep problems
- sugar craving
- fatty acid deficiencies
- vitamin and mineral deficiencies
- muscle pain

As we will see, conventional medicine finds it difficult to believe that candida can cause all these different symptoms. Many doctors feel that it is used as a vague, 'catch-all' diagnosis when the practitioner cannot find out what is really going on in a patient. They are suspicious of a diagnosis which is often arrived at without a definite, objective laboratory test to confirm it and which may involve a vulnerable individual in a complex programme of treatment that will probably last many months and will almost certainly involve them in costs of hundreds of pounds for natural (or otherwise) medicines. In response, natural health practitioners argue that there *is* a valid laboratory test for candida overgrowth now available, which, when backed up with simple tests for allied conditions such as 'leaky gut syndrome' and the involvement of the adrenal glands, can give a reliable and objective picture of what is going on. It is true to say, however, that not as many practitioners are using these tests as should be.

Opinions also differ about the best way to treat candida. Conventional medicine has potent anti-fungal drugs in its armoury. However, many therapists believe that these may not be effective against the entrenched fungal form of candida and that because they do not fully eradicate the condition, their use is actually encouraging the development of strains that are resistant to medication.

Dealing with systemic candida overgrowth is not

always easy. However, since the early 1980s, when Alabama physician Dr C. Orian Truss and his colleague Dr William Crook first began to publicize its unsuspected role in so many health problems, a basic anti-candida protocol has been tried, tested and refined. It is continually revised in the light of new research and as natural health companies develop new natural anti-fungals and other nutritional and herbal aids.

Much of this information is anecdotal and has not been subjected to the medical gold-standard of the double-blind trial. However, there is much in traditional medical practice that is similarly untested. Candida treatment is ahead of academic research. It is driven by feedback from people who have successfully re-established the internal ecological balance necessary to stop the condition causing problems. This is not necessarily a bad thing, in fact it has advantages as well as disadvantages, as will become clear in this book. But if you suspect that you are suffering from candida overgrowth it is something you need to be aware of. Nobody has all the answers yet. There are many different approaches to treatment and it seems that no one method is guaranteed to work for everyone; you will need to mix and match to suit your individual situation.

If you are contemplating self-diagnosis and self-treatment, first do try to get an objective assessment either from an experienced practitioner or through contact with a self-help group. It could save a lot of time and money.

This book aims to give you a good start to learning how to get candida back in balance. It suggests when to use conventional medicine and when using complementary and alternative therapies, particularly nutritional therapy, may be your best option. It is not intended to be the last word on the subject, so please make full use of the resources listed at the back of the book.

CHAPTER 1

What is candida?

Candida albicans is a an old friend. One of around 80 different types of candida, it is present in most of us from birth. If we do not pick it up from our mothers during the journey down the birth canal, it will get to us like other micro-organisms as our birth helpers and proud parents touch and kiss us.

Candida is dimorphic, which literally means it has two forms. It is a yeast that also has a fungal form and is often referred to as a yeast-like fungus. Normally it causes us few problems. Most healthy, symptom-free people will have it somewhere about their persons – on their hands, in their hair, in their mouths. Although it can exist on the skin and in the hair its ideal living conditions are warm, moist and dark places, such as the gut, the vagina, the mouth and the mucous membranes of the tubes connecting the nose and lungs. Even here it is usually easily contained by billions of helpful bacteria that successfully compete for both living space and nutrients. If we have a healthy immune system, we also automatically keep candida in balance through the activation of specialist white blood cells to destroy it.

In everyday medical practice, candida overgrowth is termed candidiasis (pronounced 'candy-die-a-sis'), candidosis or thrush, and sometimes also as moniliasis, from the original name for this type of fungus. Doctors usually make a preliminary diagnosis from the appearance of tell-tale white patches on the tongue or genitals, accompanied by a discharge a bit like soft cheese. It can sometimes also affect the lining of the heart and be a factor in the inflammatory condition known as endo-carditis.

Although candida, as a typical yeast, is literally every-where – in the air, in the soil and on food as well as on everyone around us – in medical terms candidiasis is seen as the result of an infection. It is true that thrush may be sexually transmitted, thereby reaching parts it might not normally reach; but we are also quite likely to 'infect' ourselves by transferring Candida when we scratch and rub our ears or nose, for instance.

While there is good research evidence and clinical experience to support the idea of treating thrush as a purely local problem, confined to the mouth or the geni-tals, and that a short and simple treatment with a prescribed anti-fungal drug will often do the job, it appears that this traditional candida picture is changing. More and more people are finding that their candida does not go away so easily and are wondering whether it might have something to do with their general state of health. If they are suffering particularly from digestive problems, allergies or abdominal bloating or are tired all the time, they may well suspect that they are suffering not just from a quick attack of thrush but from a con-tinuous, long-term overgrowth of candida that is spreading all over the place.

Most medical practitioners are not sympathetic to this view, since they are taught that this whole-body, or sys-temic, level of infection is rare and that when it does occur it is an acute and potentially fatal condition. Indeed they may have encountered people with this degree of candida during their training in hospitals.

This concept of infection may be another reason why most medical practitioners are reluctant to take on the idea of systemic candida overgrowth. The view that most disease is caused by germs, invading micro-organisms that can overpower us unless we are suitably defended with drugs, vaccinations and the like, leaves little room for any suggestion that disease may also arise from within. But after all, give yeasts and fungi the conditions they need to grow and they will do just that. An old naturopathic saying is 'Flies do not cause dustbins'. In other words, you may create conditions favourable for disease to occur by the choices you make about what you eat and how you live your life. If you treat your body as a dustbin – and never 'empty' it by having stress-free periods or times when you eat and drink healthily – then its hardly surprising if 'flies' are attracted and start breeding and spreading disease. It is little use then attacking the flies – the bacteria, viruses or fungi you have invited in – and blaming them for causing the 'dustbin' – your poor state of health. In this view, the emphasis is on the conditions inside our bodies. If they are favourable for candida, then it starts to grow. If they are unfavourable then even if we are 'infected' it will not grow. The advantage of looking at things in this way is that it is empowering: it gives you plenty of opportunity to take positive action to change things for the better.

Faced with obvious signs of candida in the mouth or vagina, the question needs to be asked where it is coming from. Is it really just something that has been picked up like any other infection – which is quite possible – or is it spreading from inside? Is it just a dirty sink that needs a quick swill down with bleach, or do you need to treat the drains? Different systems of medicine reach different conclusions at that point. However, it is worth observing that researchers at Michigan State University investigating women with recurrent vaginal candidiasis (thrush), concluded that every woman with a vaginal yeast infection has an 'intestinal reservoir' of yeasts overgrowing in her digestive tract.

Some commentators believe that the medical profession as a whole just does not want to know about chronic candida overgrowth because there is evidence to suggest that more often than not it is directly caused by conventional medical treatment with antibiotics and corticosteroids, and as a side-effect of the contraceptive pill. Because hormonal changes during the menstrual cycle and pregnancy affect the balance of bacteria in the gut, because of its association with the pill and because women tend to receive more medical treatment and more antibiotics than men, candida overgrowth is more common in women than in men. Ironically, in men infected with HIV, the virus associated with AIDS, some of the symptoms of candida, such as chronic fatigue and recurrent bouts of fever, may be mistakenly attributed to HIV.

As we shall see, thanks largely to the use of antibiotics and to diets rich in sugar, Candida nowadays often finds conditions that are absolutely ideal for it to flourish. Antibiotics depress the immune system, which also takes a battering from recreational drugs and the increasing amounts of nutrient-poor junk foods, such as alcohol, caffeine and sugar, round which our modern lifestyle seems to revolve. Add in immune systems that are not functioning too well, or that are temporarily depressed, and it is easy to see why researchers believe that candida has never had it so good. The result, they believe, is that we are seeing an under-reported explosion in a new type of candida condition which is being variously referred to as chronic candidiasis, yeast syndrome, chronic candida syndrome and candida-related complex (CRC).

This type of systemic overgrowth is termed 'bloodstream infection' by the multicentre researchers of the Candida Adherence Mycology Research Unit. They report that it increased by 219–487 per cent between 1980 and 1989. In the USA these yeast-type fungi now account for 10 per cent of all the infections picked up by patients while in hospitals. This rate of infection now equals one of the most common – and potentially fatal – micro-organisms, E coli, and has overtaken cases of Klebsiella, a bacterium that can cause pneumonia and respiratory infections. Indeed, candida is the fourth leading cause of hospital infections. According to researcher Dr Jim

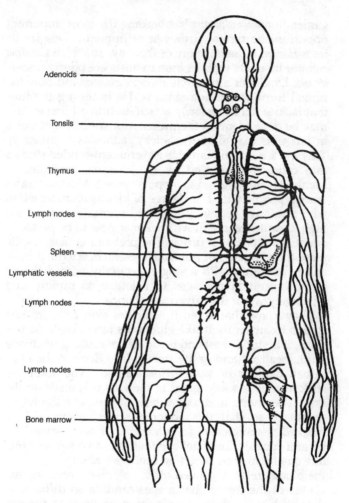

Fig. 1 The immune system

Cutler, '*Candida albicans* has become the most important opportunistic fungal pathogen of humans.' Despite its importance, he says, many of the ways in which *Candida albicans* interacts with its human hosts are poorly understood. Dr Cutler's research aims to understand how the fungal form of candida spreads. He is testing the idea that it does not necessarily attach itself to all tissues and may be dependent on the presence of specific molecules in our cells that allow its 'sticky' adhesins to attach it. This work is one of many US government-funded studies into candida supported by the National Institutes of Mental Health in a bid to stop its spread. Mortality rates among people with this degree of bloodstream infection who also have seriously impaired immune systems are high, despite treatment with what appear to be perfectly adequate anti-fungal drugs. The problem is that despite more than 20 years of published research, scientists have still to come up with a single, generally agreed theory of how candida manages to colonize so rapidly and effectively when it is given the chance.

They know that when it colonizes skin cells, its first step is to attach itself like glue to its target cells. At this stage, it is still a yeast and is capable of causing relatively mild, localized and easily treated infections of the skin, throat, bladder or vagina, for instance. The ability to stick to cells is a key factor in the way it spreads on the skin. They hope to discover how to mobilize the host's resistance so that this adherence mechanism will be blocked, leaving candida vulnerable to being wiped up by anti-fungals. They believe that the same sort of glue-like quality may be critical in candida's ability to get into the bloodstream and head off to colonize target organs.

One of the things that makes candida so difficult to deal with is its ability to change from yeast to fungus. One of the ways it gets through 'barriers' such as mucous membranes which are specifically designed to hinder micro-organisms, is that having locked on to cells, in its fungal form it puts down root-like 'threads' which use their own enzymes to dissolve the proteins that hold cells together. They can thus invade cells in search of nutrients and burrow between them, creating spaces in which candida can reproduce or maybe even 'hide' if defensive immune system cells are on the prowl.

Once the deep-rooted fungal form of candida is established it can become extremely difficult to eradicate. As we shall see, it appears that many anti-fungal treatments either are not able to penetrate deeply enough to clear it totally, or they simply miss it altogether. Meanwhile, it produces toxins that help it survive and alter the immediate environment so that it can carry on colonizing. When it has punched microscopic holes in the wall of the intestine or other membrane, the toxic by-products it produces when it ferments sugars and the other poisons it produces are no longer isolated in the gut but can be absorbed into the blood. One of the body's responses is to make antibodies to candida, which in turn help to trigger an immune system attack on it. With candida in the system and with other yeasts in the diet, there follows what amounts to a continual immune system 'red alert', with hypersensitivity and its attendant chronic inflammation as part of daily life.

In effect, candida can cause a three-stage reaction: unpleasant local infections, deeper disturbances affecting the digestion and metabolism due to its presence in the gut, and an allergic or allergic-type response. This is why it can be responsible for such an enormously wide range of symptoms, from thrush and skin rashes to chronic fatigue and digestive problems, including pre-menstrual difficulties, depression, poor memory and lack of concentration as well as other mental and emotional problems, mood swings, confusion, recurrent herpes infection, joint and muscle pains, food cravings (particularly for bread, sweets and perhaps alcohol), indigestion and food sensitivities and intolerances (not to mention full-blown allergies), and sensitivity to moulds, dampness and environmental pollution (including cigarette smoke).

Research in the UK and at the National Institutes of Mental Health in the USA has suggested an explanation for candida's effects on mind and mood. Incomplete protein-breakdown products, if absorbed because of the fungal form's roots threading through the gut wall, may act like endorphins, the body's natural pain-killing chemicals (also known to be released during periods of heavy exercise, giving rise to the so-called 'runner's high'). These chemicals can change one's mood and affect the mind, memory and behaviour. Endorphins are hormones, the body's chemical messengers, released by the master gland of our endocrine system, the pituitary, directly into the bloodstream, and have only relatively recently begun to be researched. Some scientists suggest that they are used by the body to regulate energy output and conservation. It is already clear, according to Dr Ernest Rossi, that they can affect the way we respond to stress, pain, mood, appetite and performance. They have been dubbed 'exorphins'.

As is usual with candida, there are different opinions about what goes on with this fungal form. One school of thought believes it is a natural evolutionary stage in candida's life-cycle and occurs when conditions are right. Others believe that the organism is forced into its fungal form when conditions are bad; it puts down roots in order to find food or space to expand.

There is a difference of opinion too about 'leaky gut syndrome'. This condition is important in the candida story, because when, for whatever reason, candida goes into overdrive in the small intestine, its roots drill holes in the walls of the intestinal tract that are large enough to allow partly digested particles of food to leach into the bloodstream, along with toxins and bits of yeast. This provokes an immune response, and from that point on the immune system is primed to react whenever traces of those 'invaders' are encountered in the future. As these errant particles include common foods, this could lead to unwelcome reactions or, in the worst cases, to a constant stressful state of biochemical 'red alert'. Many practitioners believe that this is one of the major causes of food allergies and intolerances.

However American naturopathic physician Michael Murray warns that candida is not the only cause of a leaky gut, or increased gastrointestinal permeability to give it its official name, and that this can give rise to many classic symptoms of candida overgrowth, but with no overgrowth happening. This may not be appreciated by many practitioners attempting to treat candida, while others do not accept the importance of leaky gut syndrome and will treat candida without doing anything to help heal the gut.

So, is there a way of telling if you have thrush or a more widespread overgrowth of candida? As far as objective laboratory tests go, there is again controversy in that conventional practitioners tend to rely completely upon standard tests, although such tests are not always of that much use. Standard medical tests such as checking a stool sample may not provide much information beyond the fact that candida is present, which is not very helpful, as it will most likely be present in healthy people's stools as well. This test may show whether your stool contains unusually large amounts, but it may not say whether these are the yeast form or the fungal form, or whether it is invasive or in balance. Experienced practitioners have found that a battery of different tests is necessary to get a true picture of what is going on. These may include allergy tests and adrenal function tests. Dr Murray, for example, uses a comprehensive stool and digestive analysis (CDSA) profile that looks for the presence of beneficial bacteria in the gut, as well as metabolic and digestive markers to differentiate between candida overgrowth and, for instance, leaky gut syndrome that is independent of candida.

Yeast Screen-Candascan is a stool culture test that detects all types of yeast overgrowth, not just candida, and it can be used to establish where the overgrowth is taking place. Employed along with a Serum Candida Antigen test, a urine test for leaky gut and a test that gives a measure of how much the adrenal glands are under stress, this battery of investigations can give a good picture of whether candida overgrowth is present and just how bad it is.

Given the complexity of the testing required, many practitioners, and individual patients, usually arrive at their diagnosis of systemic candida overgrowth by using checklists of symptoms and a questionnaire that also assesses the individual's exposure to common risk factors. Typical key questions are:

- Have you ever taken a course of antibiotics for one month or more, or have you ever taken several courses of antibiotics in the course of a year?
- Have you ever been treated with steroids?
- Have you used the contraceptive pill?
- Have you been pregnant more than once?
- Have you been treated with immunosuppressive medication?
- Have you had thrush more than once?
- Have you had fungal infections of the nails or skin, including athlete's foot, ringworm or 'jock itch'?
- Do you suffer from allergies?
- Have you had recurrent or persistent cystitis, vaginitis or prostatitis?
- Do you suffer regularly from pre-menstrual syndrome?
- Do you regularly suffer:
  bloating
  diarrhoea
  constipation
  headaches
  depression
  fatigue
  poor memory
  impotence

    lack of sexual desire
    feelings of unreality, feeling 'spaced out'
    muscular aches and pains (for no apparent cause)
    pains and swelling in joints (for no apparent cause)
    erratic vision or visual disturbances?

- Are symptoms worse on damp, muggy days or in mouldy places?
- Do you crave sweet foods, bread or alcohol?
- Are you sensitive to tobacco smoke, perfumes, insecticides and other chemicals?

If patients answer 'yes' to many of these questions, particularly to those relating to antibiotic and other drug use, they may well be likely to have candida. As a final check, they are typically asked to also check a 'minor' symptom list; if several of these symptoms are also present then candida overgrowth is probable:

- persistent drowsiness
- lack of co-ordination
- mood swings
- loss of balance
- frequent rashes
- mucus in stools
- belching and gas
- bad breath
- dry mouth or throat
- haemorrhoids
- rash or blisters in the mouth
- post-nasal drip
- nasal congestion or discharge
- heartburn and indigestion
- ear pain or deafness
- recurrent ear infections
- frequent or urgent urination

The more symptoms are being experienced and the more severe they are, the more likely it is that candida could be a major problem; the practioner is looking for a collection of signs, symptoms and risk factors, not just a few isolated ones.

Most practitioners attempting to treat candida use variations of this questionnaire, the original of which seems to have been put together by the pioneering Dr Bill Crook in his 1983 book *The Yeast Connection*.

Do remember that the practical treatment of candida overgrowth is in advance of research. It is an area where definitive answers are not always available – where, for example, it is not always possible to explain why some treatments may work well for one person and not for another. There is a real worry that many people have convinced themselves that they have candida and are treating themselves for it, while the problem is really something else, such as a relatively simple food intolerance, or a more 'mechanical' musculo-skeletal problem, for instance, which might be better addressed by therapies such as osteopathy, chiropractic or other forms of bodywork.

A good place to start is with the questionnaire given above. If you have a lot of the risk factors and many of the symptoms seem to apply to you, you may want to try the basic anti-candida diet for one month while taking one of the recommended natural anti-fungals (*see* chapter 5). If nothing happens – if you feel no better and no worse – there is every possibility that you do not have candida. If necessary, get professional advice from a practitioner used to dealing with the condition and contact a self-help group for information on the latest developments.

If you do have health problems that you suspect are due to candida, do not let anyone put you off investigating it and treating it thoroughly. Dr Robert Cathcart, an American doctor specializing in nutritional treatment, is one of many who feel that *Candida albicans* is one of our century's most serious conditions. He says:

The allergy connection

There is strong link between candida and allergies; in fact candida symptoms were originally thought to be entirely due to an allergic reaction to the appearance of candida in the intestines. Research now seems to support the idea that while this may happen, a far bigger problem is that candida overgrowth may cause:

- an overall increase in sensitivity to yeasts, moulds and fungi
- intolerances and sensivities to many different foods and everyday chemicals such as perfumes and household cleaners

Allergy specialist Dr James Braly, the founder of Optimum Health Laboratories in California, says of candida: 'Its symptoms often mimic those of food allergy and because the two are sometimes interrelated . . . must be treated together.'

Candida itself produces over 70 toxins. As if these were not enough to cause a constant state of 'red alert' in the immune system, it can also cause microscopic holes in the wall of the intestines which allow undigested molecules of food to get into the blood. The results can be a stream of symptoms similar to food allergies, exhaustion and an inability of the immune system to be able to turn its attentions to the candida itself. This is what is termed a compromised immune system – one that is already 'stretched', and so is unable to deal with everyday bugs when they happen along, with the result that the patient may go down with recurrent colds and flu attacks.

True food allergies are in fact quite rare. They are usually immediate and dramatic, which is why they can be identified with skin-scratch testing: if someone is allergic to a substance he or she will react with an immediate swelling, a weal, when minute particles of it are scratched into the tissue just under your skin.

Far more common, according to the latest thinking of

specialists like Dr Braly, are delayed-response food allergies, or intolerances, which involve a different pathway of the immune system. In most cases of classic food allergies, symptoms such as inflammation, asthma, hay fever, hives, sneezing and so on, start as soon as one is exposed to even a tiny amount of the food or substance one is sensitive to. In contrast, in delayed reactions, the amount of food involved varies enormously. And, whether or not there is a reaction at all may also depend on what patients eat the offending substance with, and the amount of stress they are under when they eat it, as Dr Braly explains in his book *Dr Braly's Optimum Health Program* (Times Books, 1985).

However, the key fact to remember is that with these type of intolerances, one usually does not see an immediate reaction. Symptoms such as bloating, skin rashes, headache and fatigue may arise hours after eating the suspect food; sometimes they will not develop until up to 48 hours later, as has been proved by research with migraine sufferers. Obviously, this makes it difficult to track down what food or chemical is causing the reaction.

The good news is that you do not even have to start this sort of hunt. Experience shows that in most people, this hypersensitivity response corrects itself as the candida population in the gut declines and the intestine is healed.

Candida should be sought and treated. It should be emphasized to patients that they owe it to themselves and society to treat the candida consistently because of the possibility of breeding resistant strains.

Part of the problem now emerging with bacteria that are resistant to antibiotics is that many patients given antibiotics do not take the the full course; they stop taking the tablets as soon as they start to get better, which enables the bacteria to bounce back, having received just enough antibiotic to get used to it.

Preliminary research suggests that candida can be

transmitted from one person to another through physical contact. In Japan, doctors believe that *Candida albicans* is routinely passed on in this way, and may also be picked up through contaminated food. The UK's *National AIDS Manual* warns:

> As some strains can be resistant to anti-fungal treatment, this raises the possibility that drug-resistant strains could be passed on to somebody who has never received anti-fungal treatment.

Dr Cathcart says that if tests cannot confirm that people have candida, then sensitivities to the condition should be suspected. Treatment to correct the bacterial balance in the gut and heal any damage to its lining should be considered. There is a high incidence of food and chemical sensitivities associated with candida, he says, and it must be suspected whenever such sensitivities are discovered.

CHAPTER 2

What goes on in the gut?

We do not normally think about our digestive system unless something goes wrong with it. But in order to understand how a candida overgrowth is able to wreak the havoc that it does, we need to look inside – or rather 'outside'. After all, our digestive system is essentially a long tube running from mouth to anus. It is designed to keep everything that is inside it *outside* our bodies until it has been broken down and chemically altered – digested – into an acceptable form and a suitable size to be absorbed into the blood or lymph, which then carries it to where it is needed. You cannot get the energy in a sandwich straight to your muscles, for example. First your teeth break the sandwich down a bit, while digestive enzymes in your saliva start to disintegrate it chemically; the process goes on and on with the pieces of food becoming smaller and smaller, until they are minute enough to be allowed from the 'outside' into your blood. At the same time, everything is checked for safety.

To this end, the digestive system is lined with specialized mucous membranes and protected with a veritable armoury of special features, from the bug-destroying acid in the stomach to the muscular mobility of areas like the small intestine. And playing a very important role in keeping us safe from the ravages of bacteria, viruses, parasites and their associated poisonous by-products are colonies, billions strong, of helper bacteria.

These micro-organisms are just like us. They have found a nice environmental niche for themselves and have evolved to make the most of it. When we look at what goes on in the gut, we need to be ecologists and start thinking in terms of habitats, population densities and survival strategies. What we have inside us is in many ways as complex as any other delicately balanced natural habitat: as with a coral reef or a rainforest, for the system to continue to flourish, natural checks and balances must enable different life-forms to coexist.

There are around 400 different species of bacteria spread from mouth to anus throughout our gastrointestinal tract. The bacteria in our large intestine weigh around 3lb, large enough really to be considered an organ in their own right. In fact, although the liver is considered to be the body's busiest metabolic factory, some experts say that the metabolic activity of the gut bacteria is potentially equal.

These bacteria are busy. They help complete the digestive process by slowing the rate at which food leaves the stomach, breaking down parts of protein and carbohydrates and certain types of sugars and fats, including, some researchers believe, cholesterol. They synthesize vitamins, mainly in the large intestine, including B1, B2, B6, B12, folic acid, biotin, niacin, pantothenic acid and vitamin K (the B vitamin biotin stops candida yeast being transformed into the fungal form). Preliminary evidence also suggests that they probably also improve the availability of minerals and stimulate the immune system.

The bacteria also have a protective role, increasing our resistance to other bugs, even virulent food-poisoning bacteria. One of the ways they do this is by producing natural antibiotics such as acidophilin, which is effective against an enormous number of potentially disease-causing organisms. By converting lactose (milk sugar) into lactic acid, bacteria also keep the environment of the intestine slightly acidic, which is unfavourable to candida as well as other disease-causing agents such as cholera, salmonella and giardia.

One study showed how a daily supplement of *Lacto-*

bacillus acidophilus, the prime helper bacteria, protected people against 'traveller's tummy' during trips to Nepal, Mexico and Guatemala. Dr Keith Schnert, in collaboration with Augsburg College in Minneapolis, recruited 70 travellers who were given two capsules a day of acidophilus. Only two reported any diarrhoea or digestive problems, compared with the expected 14–20.

An established and healthy gut flora, with its several indigenous species, has other simpler ways of keeping candida in balance: it fills the available living space and uses up the sugars that candida would otherwise take advantage of.

If candida is given free run of the intestinal environment when other more 'friendly' bacteria have been wiped out by antibiotics, for instance, it is quick to take advantage. The yeast proliferates and infects more and more of our cells, causing them to die off. German biologist Joachim Hartmann, who has studied the candida life-cycle, suggests that it is the breaking up of cells, releasing their content of water, energy and other nutrients, that stimulates candida to transform itself from yeast to fungus. Another theory is that it starts to put down its roots in a search of sugar and/or space, which would hold true whether candida is suffering shortages because of its own population explosion or whether it is being starved by a strict diet. It may be, however, that it starts to change as soon as there is a deficiency of the factors – such as the B vitamin biotin – that normally stop it.

The main breeding ground where all this happens is the small intestine, into which the stomach empties, and further down the large intestine or colon. There are relatively few bacteria in the small intestine (which is technically divided into three parts – the duodenum, jejenum and ileum) and they are dominated by the lactic acid 'family' such as *Lactobacillus acidophilus* and *Lactobacillus casei*. The small intestine is fed with the contents of the stomach. When stomach acid is sufficiently high,

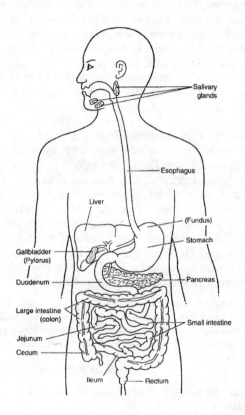

Fig. 2 The digestive system

few disease-causing organisms get through. Similarly, the acid from the stomach is needed to stimulate the pancreas, lower down the digestive chain, to produce alkaline juices. This change from acid to alkaline enables pancreatic enzymes to take over the digestion of food in the small intestine after it has left the stomach, and can also affect the bacterial balance, since the 'friendly' bacteria normally resident in this part of the intestine cannot survive an acid environment. The mobility of the small intestine moves food through relatively quickly, making it difficult for food-poisoning bacteria to attach themselves to the walls and cause trouble. However, we absorb most of the nutrients from our food in the small intestine, so if anything interferes with its normal function the potential for disease is high.

In the large intestine, the flow of digesting food is slower and, as a result, there is a massive growth of bacteria, but only those that are able to survive totally without oxygen. Different species dominate here: the helpful *Bifido* bacteria and the neutral *Bacteroides*.

According to Dr Nigel Plummer, a microbiologist and biotechnologist specializing in this area, the differences in the sizes of population are staggering:

> In the normal stomach there is likely to be less than one hundred organisms per gram of contents. In the small intestine it will range from ten thousand to one million per gram, and in the colon it will rise to a staggering one thousand billion per gram.

> (*BioMed Newsletter*, no. 10, 1984)

About half the weight of our faecal material is comprised of bacteria.

When we take antibiotics by mouth, they pass through the stomach and into the small intestine, where they are absorbed into the bloodstream. Dr Plummer describes what happens next:

> While the dissolved antibiotic is in the small intestine waiting to be absorbed, it is at a concentration far in excess

of its systemic working concentration (bloodstream concentration). This means that the population of micro-organisms in the small intestine is exposed to a super concentrated solution of antibiotics and very few of these micro-organisms survive.

The effect of common antibiotics such as oxy-tetracycline, tetracycline and ampicillin on *Lactobacillus acidophilus* is dramatic: it is wiped out.

Conversely, once the antibiotic is in the bloodstream it is effectively diluted and becomes further diluted as it is distributed throughout the various organ and tissue types of the body. Thus the large intestine and its microflora are only exposed to a very dilute level of antibiotics compared to the upper small intestine. Moreover, the mass of bacteria in the large intestine is so vast that antibiotics have little effect on the total number.

So as a result of antibiotics, the small intestine is virtually stripped of its microflora, and loses all their metabolic and protective functions. In contrast, the large intestine still holds a thriving population of microbes. 'These will then migrate into the small intestine where the ecological niche is now available for colonization.'

Unfortunately, the antibiotic-altered environment of the small intestine in this condition usually favours the growth of organisms, such as faecal streptococci, which are undesirable in large numbers and can also help to push out the 'friendly' bacteria that help keep candida in check.

Dr Plummer reports:

Occasionally, but more often than is generally recognized, the recolonization of the small intestine can take place while the antibiotic is being used. This is the situation where yeast species – usually *Candida albicans* – become established in the small intestine, as a result of having been unaffected by antibiotics. Once established, yeasts are very difficult to dislodge.

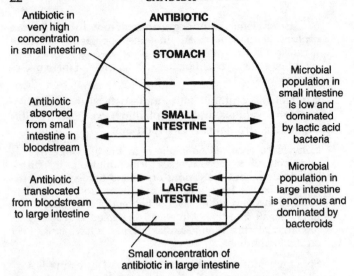

Fig. 3 How antibiotics affect bacteria in the gut (courtesy of Dr Nigel Plummer and *BioMed Newsletter*)

It is important to remember that candida is not supposed to be dominant in the small intestine, and for good reason, as it competes with us for the food we are trying to digest. Like any good yeast, candida gets hold of sugar and starts 'digesting' it, producing gas and aldehyde, a type of alcohol. The result in our intestines is bloating, rumbling and wind. Yeasts also feed on protein, producing potentially toxic chemicals called vasoactive amines. They are called 'vasoactive' because they affect the muscles controlling (vaso)constriction and (vaso)dilation of blood vessels. According to naturopathic physician Dr Michael Murray, amines contribute to leaky gut syndrome, as well as causing abdominal pain and changing the way the gut moves spontaneously to help keep disease-causing micro-organisms from colonizing.

At some point, candida changes from its mild-mannered yeast form into a disease-causing fungus, interfering with metabolism and digestion, destroying cells and damaging tissues such as the gut wall, and eventually it may cause organs to become inefficient. According to Dr Pavel Yutsis, reporting in a 1992 paper presented to the American Academy of Environmental Medicine:

> Extremely potent toxins known as canditoxins will be released and a minimum of 79 known chemical substances will challenge the human body to produce identifiable antigens.

An antigen is a substance that can trigger and get involved in an immune response. This could be seen as a major stress to the immune system, especially as there are more than 80 candida strains, of which *Candida albicans* is one, implying that as candida begins to multiply, our immune system could be being asked to produce a response to thousands of different chemicals.

Hartmann says:

> Strictly speaking, candida yeasts are not considered 'pathogenic' since they can't trigger an infection in normally healthy people. Some sort of change in the 'ecology' of the body must first occur before a candida colonization with disease symptoms can make its appearance. However, even minor deviations of the body's physiology, its defensive capability and the internal flora can suffice. The extent of the 'terrain' changes determines the severity of the candidiasis.

The big problem seems to be that when the 'terrain' has been altered, whether by antibiotics or other drugs, combined with stress, a high-sugar diet and possibly the contraceptive pill as well, candida seems to be able to grow back more quickly than the protective bacteria. The conventional belief is that after antibiotics your normal flora eventually just re-establishes itself, but there is little convincing evidence that this happens.

A more likely scenario is that antibiotics are just one

factor in a massive alteration of the environment inside the body. Even with a candida-favouring diet and a certain amount of stress, the colonies of protective bacteria are large enough to dominate the environment physically and chemically. But when antibiotics wipe them out, candida has room to colonize, has access to the nutrients, chiefly sugar, it needs, and is no longer affected by the acids and anti-microbial chemicals which would normally be being produced by 'friendly' bacteria.

By the time a course of antibiotics is stopped the damage has been done. Research does show that whatever organisms are then dominant, stay dominant. Many people with candida have a history of not one course of antibiotics, but frequent, long-term treatment. This means that the condition has been given the best possible chance to become firmly entrenched.

CHAPTER 3

Causes and risk factors

Candida needs three things to start making a nuisance of itself: somewhere to live, a steady supply of food and a window of opportunity where it is relatively free from surveillance or attack by our immune system. Unfortunately, our modern lifestyle seems to fulfil all candida's basic requirements.

Antibiotics

Most researchers agree that the use of antibiotics is the single biggest factor in the emergence of candida as a chronic overgrowth problem. Antibiotics drastically alter the microecology of the gut which, as we saw in the previous chapter, is vital for good health and for preventing candida and other opportunistic parasites from causing trouble. Candida is able to grow back more quickly than our protective helper bacteria because the average diet, rich in refined sugar and high in carbohydrates (which are complex forms of sugar), favours the growth of yeast.

Naturopathic physician Dr Joseph Pizzorno comments: 'Candida overgrowth is an all too common result of antibiotics given to hospitalized patients.' In his book *Total Wellness* he reports on a 1993 study which found that every single one of 55 patients admitted to one hospital's casualty department was given broad-spectrum antibiotics. Blood tests showed that 67 per cent of them developed candida overgrowth. The researchers also found that immune-system white blood cells from patients with overgrowth were not able to stop candida growing as effectively as white blood cells from those patients who had remained clear of candida.

In other words, when patients receive antibiotics, the level of candida in their intestines increases so much and the intestines become so damaged, that pieces of the candida leak into their blood and inhibit the function of their immune systems.

Pneumonia and tuberculosis are making a comeback. Even hospitals are struggling to keep under control bacteria that are immune to almost all the drugs that used to stop them dead. Meanwhile, there has been a steady increase in food poisoning – from only 1,000 reported cases in 1980 to current totals of around 40,000–50,000 cases a year in the UK alone. If one takes into account those cases which are not reported, but are dealt with by doctors or self-treated, there are probably now around 500,000 a year.

According to a World Health Organisation (WHO) report, the bugs are developing resistance to antibiotics faster than drug companies can develop new ones. 'This resistance problem is one that I think is going to be a major plague for the coming century,' predicts Ralph Henderson, WHO's Assistant Director.

Scientists fear that we are about to return to the days before penicillin, when routine infections were killers. Babies, children and the elderly are particularly at risk of serious long-term illness or even death. So, the 'superbugs' are coming. And there are now fears that the conventional anti-fungals used to treat candida are going to face the same problem. Dr Pavel Yutsis, an allergy specialist, says that nystatin, for instance, 'can't completely rid the body of *Candida albicans*'. Instead he feels that it may allow for the subsequent development of nystatin resistance, as the candida it fails to eradicate pass on their resistance to succeeding generations. Unfortunately, it is not just a question of getting us to stop taking antibiotics for the slightest infection. Many farm animals are regularly dosed with antibiotics, not just for infections but also as growth promoters. As a result, one strain of the food poisoning bug salmonella, for example, has already developed multiple drug resistance and has spread throughout British cattle, sheep, pigs and poultry. Scientists have already discovered this strain in humans and suspect that it was passed on in sausages, chicken or burgers. Birmingham University microbiologists have found that one in four chickens bought in British supermarkets contain food-poisoning bacteria resistant to commonly prescribed antibiotics which are similar to another drug widely used in battery farming.

Cooking does not kill all these 'superbugs' and nor does pasteurization; another microbe, suspected of causing Crohn's disease, a serious inflammatory condition of the bowel, has been found in UK shop-bought cow's milk. UK Ministry of Agriculture tests found one in 30 samples of pork and eggs contaminated with antibiotics above government safety levels. And scientists at a European seminar blamed antibiotics used by farmers for an up to 10 per cent rise in food poisoning cases. In the USA, a study at Rutgers University found that antibiotics used at levels deemed safe for human consumption by the Food and Drug Administration (FDA) increased the rate of development of resistant bacteria by 600–2,700 per cent.

Dr Peter Wilson, Lecturer in Microbiology at University College Hospital, London, has said that breaches of known safety limits were endangering the elderly, the sick and those with compromised immune systems – which, as we have seen, includes everyone with chronic candida overgrowth.

Perhaps the most worrying 'superbug' is a type of everyday *Staphylococcus*, which can cause skin infections and abscesses, and is often implicated in food poisoning. Until very recently this bug was still vulnerable to one prescription antibiotic, but a resistant strain has now been found in Japan and the USA and it is only a matter of time before it occurs in other countries. Meanwhile, in an effort to wipe out persistent 'superbug' infections, multiple antibiotic treatments are being used, often in massive doses, which is wreaking havoc on our internal bacterial ecology and paving the way for an epidemic of chronic candida overgrowth.

Other factors

To add to our discomfort, the modern lifestyle has become synonymous with stress. When we are under stress, even if we are coping well with it, we naturally produce chemicals that can depress our immune systems. Candida does not need much help on this score. Once established, it starts producing its own toxins that can protect it from being attacked by the cells of our immune system. But stress also affects the bacteria in our gut, shifting the balance in favour of disease-producing microbes and parasites such as candida. It does this because in response to stress, the normal secretions of our digestive system become more acidic and the natural movements of the gut are decreased – conditions that our helper *Lactobacillus* and *Bifido* bacteria do not like.

Another factor that may be important is the way in which we have come to rely on carbohydrates in general and wheat in particular. In evolutionary terms, wheat is a relative newcomer, appearing in our diets as a result of the agricultural revolution of some 10,000 years ago. Human physiology is still Paleolithic, virtually unchanged for around 17 million years. There is a growing amount of evidence to suggest that we have simply not had time to adapt to wheat, a suggestion that is born out by the fact that so-called 'ancient' varieties of wheat, such as spelt, are said to be better tolerated.

It may be the refining of wheat that causes the problem, or it may be the quantities in which we now

Case study: Fiona

In terms of candida risk factors, Fiona, 41, was a classic case. 'I had always had a very sweet tooth. I used to eat Mars bars, trying to get more energy. And I had a history of throat infections as a child, so I had been given a lot of antibiotics, with tetracycline as well at one point – a fairly typical picture.' She also suffered from stress.

But she successfully used an anti-candida diet and supplements to get the condition under control. She is recovering from ME (post-viral fatigue sydrome), a condition which often goes hand-in-hand with candida, and although she has not yet overcome the ME, she says she now has 'double the energy' she had originally.

Her problems seemed to start after a bout of glandular fever and a long period of stress. 'I had a host of symptoms,' she says. The worst was a persistent, constant fatigue, and a very 'foggy' head that made it extremely difficult to concentrate. A former journalist, then active in public relations, she found herself unable even to read a book or watch television without feeling exhausted. 'I couldn't do even simple tasks for more than 20 minutes.'

She began looking for effective help. She spent a lot of money on consultations but found her first nutritionally orientated doctor 'not that helpful', although she did have tests that pinpointed candida as being a problem. Fiona put herself on a no-sugar, no-yeast anti-candida diet and the doctor gave her anti-fungal drugs. She became steadily worse. After a couple of years she went to see another nutritionist who used VegaTesting, a non-invasive health evaluation system which claims to give an electrical readout of the body's systems and organs.

'She told me that I should go on an anti-candida diet, which I knew, but gave me an absolutely key piece of information and said that I *must* cut out fruit.' That proved to be a turning point. At this time she was eating three or four pieces of fruit a day, thinking that was a healthy thing to do. She cut out fruit and for the next two weeks suffered what she descriibes as 'the most incredible die-off reaction'. Although it was unpleasant, causing a variety of acute symptoms such as headaches, nausea, depression and fatigue, this reaction is what every candida sufferer hopes to provoke, as it means the condition is dying off – the side-effects are the result of a major elimination of the associated toxins, mainly through the liver, our major organ of detox-ification.

Although she felt ill, Fiona realized that this was a sign that she was on the right track. She became stricter with the diet – no sugar, no yeast, no honey or any other form of sugar, above all no fruit – and then reached another breakthrough when she was put on a really effective sup-plement regime by a third therapist. He added the basic pattern of supplements recommended later in this book – (*see* chapter 5) including a major recolonization programme with probiotics (supplements of 'friendly' bacteria) garlic, aloe vera, caprylic acid, and the plant extract combination tested by Wolverhampton University which includes oregano, clove, artemisia, ginger and borage seed oil. This doctor gave the programme an added twist by also prescri-bing a natural supplement designed to kill protozoa, a type of parasitic mico-organism that can be easily picked up from household pets or contaminated food, and which some practitioners believe is more likely to flourish in the sort of disturbed internal environment also enjoyed by candida.

This next stage of treatment took between 18 months and two years, but the discipline was worth it. 'Since taking the supplements and doing the diet my health has improved dramatically' says Fiona. 'I'm not yet fully recovered from ME, but the candida is under control. I am able to work three to four hours a day, which is a vast improvement on 20 minutes.' In fact she has the energy to keep up with research on ME as well as writing a book on yoga and fatigue.*

consume it. Wheat is everywhere, not just in bread and cakes, but is added to almost every processed food from baked beans to fish, in some form or other. Gluten, a

* *Beat Fatigue with Yoga* by Fiona Agombar is due to be published by Element in early 1999.

protein in wheat, is known to be a major irritant for people susceptible to it, affecting the folded surfaces of the intestines known as villi which enable us to absorb nutrients from food. Some researchers believe that many more people than is generally realized may be intolerant to wheat without even suspecting it. Wheat is usually top of the list of suspect foods which practitioners recommend eliminating from the diet if intolerance or allergy is suspected. But while classic food allergy to wheat is comparatively rare, far more common is a food intolerance. This is often a delayed response, occurring anything from one hour to two days or more after eating the food. It can involve many different systems of the body and cause varied psychological and physical symptoms, perhaps because its main effects are on the mucosal lining of the digestive tract, where it can cause leaky gut. The similarities with the effects of candida are obvious, and it may be that this widespread sensitivity to wheat, causing damage to the gut wall, is another important factor in preparing the ground for candida.

CHAPTER 4

Conventional medical treatments

Dealing with candida can be a complex process and the best place to start is with your regular doctor. However, you may find that he or she will not be able to supervise the whole of your treatment, or may be unsympathetic to the idea of systemic candida overgrowth. As it is often too complicated to deal with on your own, if you find yourself in this position it is a good idea to contact one of the organizations listed at the back of this book for help in finding an experienced complementary health practitioner.

The problem doctors seem to have is twofold. First, their training tells them that candida overgrowth is unlikely to be a serious problem unless the patient is seriously immuno-compromised. Secondly, patients come with a set of symptoms which they expect the doctor to get rid of – and quickly.

A patient with candida is unlikely to set off warning bells unless he or she is obviously at risk of being immuno-compromised. This could be because the patient is:

- under severe stress
- coping with a viral infection
- taking immuno-suppressive drugs such as steroids or antibiotics
- in the midst of intense treatment for conditions such as cancer or HIV infection.

So when a doctor examines you for candida, he or she is primarily looking for white spots or red patches and discharges in the mouth and vagina, or for an infection on your skin, hair or nails. If it is discovered you are likely to be prescribed local treatment with creams, powders or suppositories, and if these do not help, then with prescription anti-fungal drugs.

Digestive problems, chronic fatigue, brain 'fag', bloating, depression and other symptoms are extremely unlikely to be linked to candida overgrowth. As scientists are many years away from uncovering the whole picture of candida, there is some justification for this narrow view. But as there is good evidence to show that candida overgrowth routinely occurs in a large percentage of people following treatment with antibiotics, perhaps long-term antibiotic use should at least become a red flag signalling a need for further investigation.

Candida in the mouth is likely to be treated with anti-yeast agents such as mouthwashes or oral solutions of drugs like fluconazole (Diflucan), which clears it completely in about two weeks. Lozenges or syrup containing the anti-fungals nystatin or amphotericin are also used.

If the infection is considered to be more widespread, fluconazole tablets can be used, or another azole drug ketoconazole (Nizoral), which can cause side-effects such as nausea and rashes and, in trials on people with HIV and candida in the oesophagus, did not work as well.

The drawback with these treatments is threefold. First, they are essentially antibiotics and may not always leave helpful gut bacteria unharmed. Secondly, there is a danger of side-effects. Thirdly, there is a concern that they may help to breed resistant strains of candida. This is already being documented. A Norwegian study, published in 1993, showed the emergence of 12 resistant candida strains in eight people with AIDS who had been treated with fluconazole for one month or longer, sometimes self-medicating, for mouth or gullet candida. A

Duke University study also revealed 'a large group of patients' whose candida symptoms would not go despite treatment with azole drugs. Rather worryingly, the chances of resistant strains developing may be enhanced by the increasing use of these drugs prophylactically. A fluconazole drug is available over the counter in what is described as a 'new, single-capsule oral treatment for vaginal thrush'. The manufacturers suggest that women keep it on hand in the medicine cabinet to be used as soon as symptoms appear. They say: 'If you know that you always get thrush at a specific time in your cycle, then ask your doctor about using a pessary or capsule treatment at the time that you usually experience the symptoms – this can help break the vicious cycle of recurrent thrush.' Well, not really. As we have already seen (*see* page 3) research clearly indicates that women with recurrent bouts of thrush have an 'intestinal reservoir' of yeast. The reason thrush recurs is that these treatments are not dealing with it.

The pharmaceutical industry is dealing with these problems in the time-honoured way: modifying existing drugs or finding completely new formulations in an endless race to stay ahead of the bacteria's developing resistance. In the USA, a new prescription anti-fungal, terbinafine HCl may replace fluconazole.

The drawbacks of drugs have already been learned by some people in the gay community who are researching effective ways to stay healthy with or without HIV, and who have wide experience of anti-fungals and antibiotics. Rufus Dennis, writing in *Continuum* magazine, says:

> Attempting to treat it with drugs like fluconazole or nystatin is not the answer. 'They may appear to eliminate the symptoms, but it is only a temporary improvement and runs the risk of not just side-effects from the drugs but a chronic fungal condition which in the long term is much harder to treat.'

The azole drugs are valued because they are absorbed from the gut, get into the bloodstream and so treat candida wherever it is. This is why they have a risk of side-effects. In contrast, nystatin and another anti-fungal antibiotic, amphotericin, are considered to be safer because they supposedly stay in the intestines and do not get into the bloodstream. It is not clear how reliable this supposition is considering the damage candida does to the gut wall. Where systemic candida is considered life-threatening amphotericin may be given by injection, in which case it bypasses the digestive system, goes straight into the blood and is regarded as extremely toxic and potentially dangerous for the patient.

Dr William Crook, one of the pioneers of candida treatment, says that despite these drawbacks, 'The azole drugs are important, safe medications and I recommend them.' To try to stop the development of resistant strains, he recommends closer monitoring of the patient's progress. As soon as there is an improvement in symptoms, he says, the azole drugs can be tapered off or even stopped after a few weeks of treatment. In addition, he says:

> A non-absorbable anti-fungal medication could be given along with the azole medication and could be continued after the azole medication is stopped. These medications include nystatin, caprylic acid and/or citrus seed extracts.

Dr Crook believes that azole drugs should not be given on their own, but that patients should also be advised to limit sugars and simple carbohydrates in their diets, to use nutritional supplements, get psychological support and avoid chemical pollutants. Dr Robert Cathcart, suggests that supplements of vitamin C may increase the effectiveness of these medications and, at the same time, help the body deal with the side-effects (for more on this, see chapter 5).

Nystatin in powder form has become the treatment of choice for many holistically inclined doctors. 'Nystatin is arguably the safest medication to be found in the British Pharmacopoeia,' says British allergy expert Dr John Mansfield. But although he believes nystatin is the most effective medication to reduce candida colonies, other practitioners assert that it can cause toxicity problems with long-term use at high doses and, at best, gives only short-term relief. As it does not always reach deep-rooted candida, there is every chance that the condition will bounce back as soon as medication is stopped.

Many natural therapists believe that nystatin is simply unnecessary, as other anti-fungals will do the job more effectively. They argue that the reason that nystatin is relatively safe is that it is poorly absorbed. It has poor penetrating power, has to be continued for many months and even then may not totally eradicate candida. As with antibiotics, the fear is that this will lead to the development of drug-resistant strains. Some research suggests that what actually happens is that prolonged use of nystatin fosters the replacement of *Candida albicans* with another variety of candida, *tropicalis*, which is said to be highly resistant to treatment.

Naturopath Leon Chaitow, who in 1985 was the first to alert the British public to the unsuspected 'guest' in their guts, points out in the latest edition of his book *Candida albicans* that nystatin is itself yeast-based. Chaitow says:

Research at the Washington University School of Medicine shows that, ultimately, after a period of treatment, when nystatin is stopped it often results in even more colonies of yeast developing than were present before its use.

Other anti-fungal drugs, the azole preparations such as Sporanox and Diflucan, may be more effective as they are extremely well absorbed in the intestines and get into the blood, but because of this they are associated with a slight but unpredictable risk of potentially serious side-effects such as liver damage. Some practitioners will tend to use them as a last resort while monitoring with liver function tests; others say they are simply not necessary. In fact there seems to be nothing these drugs can do that cannot be achieved just as effectively using natural anti-fungals as part of a co-ordinated holistic healing plan.

Perhaps the most important thing to remember is that you need to choose a treatment that you are comfortable with. Given the drawbacks of conventional anti-fungal medication, it is probably a good idea to limit their use to what is essentially first aid. Used long-term they may have limited effectiveness against deep-rooted candida and have a risk of side-effects.

Nystatin appears to be the 'least worst' option, but it has some of the same disadvantages. Used short-term during the early stages of candida overgrowth, it may well help to check its growth. By the time candida has become established and entrenched, nystatin may only skim the surface, leaving the roots of the problem untouched.

When it comes to antibiotics, think twice about taking them. Discuss it with your regular doctor; most practitioners are aware of the problems of antibiotic overuse and will advise you whether your immediate problem is really severe enough to warrant a course. If you choose not to take antibiotics, there are plenty of natural alternatives discussed later in this book which can not only work against bacteria but also help your immune system. If you do take antibiotics – and many practitioners, including the most ardent natural therapists, agree that sometimes they are not just essential but potentially life-saving – then you can help to prevent them damaging your health in the long run by replenishing your gut with helper bacteria during and especially after your antibiotic treatment.

I hope that through reading this book you will be stimulated to explore a full holistic programme. The most comprehensive treatment protocol designed for candida overgrowth is based on a four-pronged diet and nutrition approach which we will explore in the next chapter.

CHAPTER 5

How to help yourself

Treatment with a change of diet and nutritional supplements is the cornerstone of comprehensive therapy for chronic candida overgrowth. It is not a quick and easy programme, and it is well nigh impossible to follow without support, whether this comes from an experienced practitioner, your family, a candida support group or a combination of all three. That is because, using this approach, you will be tackling the problem on several different fronts at the same time with the aim not just of treating the symptoms but of changing the ecology of your body so that, long-term, candida will cease to be a problem. To do this, the treatment has four main planks: an anti-candida diet, anti-fungal agents, probiotics and supplements to heal the gut.

An anti-candida diet

This involves cutting out sugar, refined carbohydrates and food sources of yeast to remove candida's fuel supply and stop over-reactions by the immune system. It is an essential part of the anti-candida programme. Authors and researchers Gill Jacobs and Jane McWhirter, who run candida workshops and are behind the Candida Support Network based at London's All Hallows natural health centre, found that 'the diet' is the one thing that makes everybody despondent. That seems to be because candida thrives on the things we are used to having in our diets. They include foods such as bread, which many of us are used to having every day. Bread is doubly suspect on an anti-candida diet because whole wheat contains gluten, which seems to cause digestive problems and damage to the gut in many people, and is made with yeast, which is another thing to avoid. But it is not all bad news. In fact you will find yourself discovering many new foods – you will undoubtedly become a regular at your health store rather than the supermarket – and putting a much greater emphasis on foods like fresh, unprocessed vegetables, which have many benefits for your health.

The other good news is that a strict diet does not last for ever. It is impossible to say how long you will need to keep to it, but it will probably be a minimum of six months and may be as long as 18–24 months, as long as you are following the rest of the anti-candida programme. The exact length of time depends on the response you get and the speed of your recovery. However, as soon as you feel that your candida is beginning to be under control, as some of your symptoms begin to clear, you can ease up on the diet and allow some of the banned foods back occasionally. After recovery, if there are favourite foods you want back in your diet, but you are concerned that they will trigger candida, then you can use them sparingly – perhaps as 'rotated' foods (*see* box on pages 43–44).

As well as cutting out the foods which are known to favour candida, you will also need to avoid foods to which you may be allergic or intolerant, as eating these adds to the strain on your immune system and may well interfere with the healing of the gut (*see* box on pages 43–44).

You should eat more:

- **Fresh, unprocessed vegetables**. Cook your vegetables gently, preferably lightly steaming them, and if your digestion can cope with it, eat around half of them raw. Avoid mushrooms, as these are also fungi and many people with candida are sensitive to them (they are also a source of moulds); potatoes may cause problems to some people as well, due to moulds.

- **Whole grains**. Millet and brown rice are favourites. Quinoa and buckwheat (actually not wheat at all) may also be well tolerated. Other grains, such as wheat, oats, rye and barley contain gluten which may cause problems. Most people seem to find that wheat gives them most problems but can tolerate a little rye and barley and occasional oats. Corn does not contain gluten, but it is not only commonly implicated in allergies and intolerances, but is routinely avoided because of a high mould content. Instead of your usual bread you can normally have yeast-free alternatives, soda breads, sprouted breads and many speciality breads such as sour-dough rye, rye crispbreads or bread made with organic spelt flour, an ancient variety of wheat used by the Romans which is better-tolerated by some people.

- **Beans and pulses**. Beans, lentils, peas and pulses are excellent foods, but perhaps not in the way most people use them – cooked, processed, stuffed full of sugar and smothered in wheat-containing sauces straight out of a can. There is an incredible variety of these foods available in health-food stores, along with plenty of ideas for cooking them. Look out for pinto beans, many varieties of lentils and split peas.

- **Nuts and seeds**. Again, get them as fresh, raw and unprocessed as possible. Peanuts and to a lesser extent hazelnuts, are common allergy foods. Buy from a store with a good turnover to avoid moulds and nuts whose natural oils have become oxidized through long storage.

- **Meat, poultry and fish**. Combining grains and pulses may mean your protein needs are met. However, if you are the type of person who does well on more protein, you might find it difficult to go without animal foods. Quite apart from considerations of animal welfare, if you are on a candida diet you have an extra reason to avoid factory-farmed and battery-bred sources, as you want to avoid residues of agricultural chemicals such as the antibiotics often used as growth promoters. So choose organically reared, free-range meat and poultry. Fish such as salmon, mackerel, herring, trout, sardines and tuna are good sources of essential fatty acids as well as protein.

- **Eggs**. If you tolerate them, they should be free-range.
- **Fruit**. Avoid fruit if your candida is severe, as it contains too much sugar, even if it is natural! Practitioners vary a lot in their recommendations here, and the exact 'prescription' depends on the individual. If you have a moderate candida problem you may get away with one or two pieces of fruit a day, and the health benefits of this nutrient-packed raw food are worth taking the risk for. Start by cutting out fruit entirely then gradually reintroduce it. Trial and error will tell you whether a daily ration of fruit encourages your candida or whether it continues to respond to treatment. If you do choose fruit, there are some rules: avoid melons because of their mould content, and avoid dried fruit such as figs, dates and raisins because of possible mould problems, but also because they are extremely concentrated sources of sugar. Another caution: because of the digestive problems which occurring with a leaky gut, many people find it valuable not to mix fruit with other foods. The theory is that this makes digestion more difficult and encourages fermentation in the gut, leading to bloating and discomfort while candida gets a good feed on undigested sugars. It is fine to eat fruit before a meal, as, on its own, it quickly passes through to the small intestine.

Foods to avoid include:

- **Yeast**. That means cutting out bread, pizza and savoury spreads.
- **Sugar**. Avoid sweets, cakes, biscuits, pastries, canned

foods, and anything with added sucrose, fructose, glucose, dextrose, lactose (that means milk), honey, molasses, or maple syrup. Yeasts love sugar; your 'helper' bacteria and your immune system do not!

- **Refined carbohydrates**. These products are usually made from what were once wholegrains which in the refining process have lost the B vitamins you need to be able to convert them to energy and also their natural fibre 'packaging', which would normally ensure that their sugar content was digested and absorbed slowly without causing large swings in your blood sugar levels. These refined carbohydrates and starches are the basis for many 'junk' and processed foods. This means avoiding white rice, and pasta, and checking labels for modified starch.

- **Fruit juices and dried fruits**. These contain far too much fruit sugar (fructose) and moulds.

- **Moulds and fungi**. Cut out mushrooms, melons, blue cheeses and black olives, and be wary about nuts, especially peanuts.

- **Alcohol**. Not only is alcohol in itself what allergy expert Dr James Braly describes as 'a combination of highly allergic substances in solution', it presents other problems. He explains:

Even at moderate levels alcohol ... leads to a 'leaky gut' – increased permeability of the mucosal lining of the small intestine – permitting the increased absorption of partially digested food molecules (and perhaps microorganisms, enterotoxins and drugs) that normally would be screened out.

When these molecules enter the bloodstream they combine with immune system markers to form immune complexes, which are involved in allergic reactions and inflammation. Candida produces its own 'raw' version of alcohol, the toxin aldehyde, a fact which has actually been successfully used in a legal defence in a drink-driving case, and you do not want to add to your detoxification burden. A study published in the *New England Society of Allergy Proceedings* showing that alcohol can promote the absorption of allergens into the system bears out Dr Braly's view. Remember also that beer and wine is fermented using yeasts, which you should be avoiding – and may be high in sugar.

For more help with foods you *can* eat and healthy alternatives to those you cannot, see 'Further reading' at the back of this book.

Food allergies and intolerances

An important additional part of the dietary approach is to identify and remove the foods which you are allergic or intolerant to and which may therefore be adding to your toxic load and provoking an immune reaction. These are often the foods we eat every day. Most of us eat from the same small selection of foods, day in, day out, and this is suspected to be a major factor in the development of food intolerances. Chimpanzees, our nearest genetic relatives still existing on a 'natural' diet, eat around 40–60 different species of food a month, averaging about 13 different foods a day: maybe we should learn from their example!

There is no need to go overboard in trying to track down your food sensitivities, as when your intestine is healed, these reactions should stop. However it may be a good idea to avoid or cut down the foods that most commonly cause problems. Dr Jim Braly's list of the foods he has found coming up again and again in thousands of allergy tests includes:

- corn
- rye
- eggs
- citrus fruit (oranges)
- white potato
- peanuts

- yeast
- milk and dairy products
- soya beans
- chocolate
- beef
- wheat
- cheese
- coffee
- tomato
- malt
- pork

If there are some foods on this list that you just cannot do without, then you can eat them less frequently. One eating pattern that has been used with success to control and prevent allergies and intolerances is the Rotation Diet, where you 'rotate' foods so that you only eat them at the most every four days. If you are rotating cheese, for example, and you eat it on a Monday, you would not eat it again until Friday, or later (*see The Rotation Diet Cookbook* under 'Further reading').

Anti-fungal agents

These directly target candida and drastically reduce its numbers or hinder its transition from yeast to fungus.

You should use the natural anti-fungals suggested here as part of a complete programme. Diet and anti-fungals alone may give poor results long-term, as they do not correct the underlying problems that allow candida to flourish.

If you get what is known as a die-off reaction, feeling worse than ever, after using anti-fungals against candida, you are feeling the effects of toxins released by the candida dying off (*see* box on page 50). It is a sign of progress, and is used by many practitioners, in the absence of a candida test result, to confirm that candida is indeed the underlying problem.

You will need to mix and match to find the preparations that do the best job for you. Those listed below are the most highly rated. There is very little clinical evidence to confirm their efficacy but they have emerged as the best remedies through a combination of reports from practitioners and patients who have used them successfully and, in many cases, from extensive laboratory testing.

Researchers have found two important benefits from using natural preparations. First, the target bacteria, viruses or candida are unlikely to be able to develop resistance against them. Antibiotic drugs are single, relatively simple chemical compounds and that is why bacteria can adapt to them so quickly, according to Dr David Hill, Senior Lecturer in Microbiology at the University of Wolverhampton. In contrast, natural oils contain many different compounds and micro-organisms cannot adapt to them all. Secondly, they do not have the same negative impact as antibiotics on the friendly bacteria we are trying to help.

The Wolverhampton scientists followed this line of reasoning and may have achieved a breakthrough with their testing of a commercial plant extract product called Candicidin, a combination of extracts of the spices oregano, clove and ginger, along with the herb artemisia and borage seed oil. Dr Hill and his team were also the first to discover that concentrated garlic oil is highly effective against bacteria. Fresh garlic was used by the Egyptians and recommended by Hippocrates in the 1st century AD to treat infections, and many garlic preparations have been clinically tested since, but this new extract is slightly more powerful – 1 teaspoonful is equivalent to 1kg (2.2lb) of fresh garlic bulbs! So far, it has inhibited every bacterium against which it has been tested. Dr Hill's work also showed that the microbes that can cause disease appear to be naturally more sensitive to garlic oil than 'friendly' bacteria.

The following are regarded as the best natural anti-fungals:

- **Garlic**. This is the simplest and some say the best; it is certainly the cheapest! Eat it raw. If you do not like the taste, use small cloves and swallow them whole. Commercial preparations of garlic are also effective. Garlic acts against bacteria and viruses as well as against candida in both its yeast and fungal forms.

- **Candicidin**. This is a combination of anti-fungal and anti-parasitic plant oils combined with essential fatty acids to help heal the gut and support the growth of helpful bacteria. It contains extracts of oregano, clove, artemisia and ginger, with borage seed oil in a base of grapeseed oil and lauric acid, a fatty acid produced from coconut. This relatively new anti-candida product is highly effective but also gentler in action than caprylic acid (*see below*), as it takes the systemic route via the bloodstream. Researchers at the University of Wolverhampton tested Candicidin against *Candida albicans* and another four of the most virulent candida strains; it outperformed other anti-fungals. Candicidin is a good anti-fungal to start with. If you need to, you can then move on to caprylic acid.

- **Caprylic acid**. Before the development of Candicidin this was the undisputed top non-prescription, natural anti-yeast anti-fungal. It comes in three different strengths so that you can minimize the die-off reaction. And you will certainly experience die-off, according to its users. Caprylic acid is a fatty acid found in coconut oil and human breast milk.

- **Olive oil**. Olive oil is not exactly an anti-fungal, but contains oleic acid which can help stop candida's transition from yeast to fungus. It must be cold-pressed, extra virgin quality.

- **Biotin**. A B vitamin that also helps stop candida changing form, biotin should be produced by your 'helper' bacteria. It is nature's way of ensuring that although dietary intake may be unreliable (biotin is water-soluble and easily lost in cooking), you will always have enough. Then along came antibiotics, with their destructive properties.

- **Berberine**. This is a natural microbe-killer that is active against a tremendous range of disease-causing bacteria, parasites and fungi, including candida. It has become a standard remedy for many naturopathic physicians treating candida overgrowth, as it also relieves diarrhoea. It also helps the immune system and the liver. Berberine is found naturally packaged in plants such as goldenseal (*Hydrastis canadensis*) and barberry (*Berberis vulgaris*).

- **Aloe vera juice**. This preparation does everything, according to its publicity. And no less an authority than the highly-acclaimed nutritional biochemist Dr Jeff Bland reports that it is a useful anti-fungal which helps re-establish a healthy bacterial balance. Be aware, however, that not all aloe vera juices are high quality. Some have lost essential ingredients in processing and some may be sweetened.

- **Grapefruit seed extract**. According to the hype, grapefruit seed extract kills all known germs and then some. Do not believe all that is said about it, however, since much of the research which is said to validate its claims actually applies to Ciba-Geigy's pharmaceutical anti-microbial Triclosan, which although extremely safe to use has not been approved for oral use in any but the smallest amounts (it is in some toothpastes and also in shampoos). That said, many people find grapefruit seed extracts an important part of their anti-candida regime and bitter herbs have long been employed in traditional Chinese medicine for their anti-fungal effects. Some practitioners even believe that it is as effective as nystatin or caprylic acid. It is claimed that it destroys candida and other parasites without affecting friendly bacteria, but there is no hard evidence to support this. Grapefruit seed extract is available in liquid form and as encapsulated powder in different strengths. You may need to experiment to find a type that works for you, as there is no standardized extract.

- **Pau d'arco**. This South American herb, also known as taheebo, is usually taken as a tea. Anecdotal evidence that it helps against candida is strong, but research is weak. As Dr Crook says:

During the past decade I have continued to get reports describing the value of this tea (as part of a yeast-control programme) even though mechanisms to explain its benefits have not been documented.

Other remedies you can try are:

- ginger root (as tea or raw slices)
- rutabaga (a type of turnip which can be eaten raw or cooked).
- horseradish
- mathake herb tea
- Tanalbit or Tanicidin (supplies tannic acid).

Nutrition and allergy specialist Dr Robert Cathcart, of Los Altos, California, a world authority on the clinical use of large doses of vitamin C, suggests that anti-fungals may work better if taken with this vitamin, as in theory they may more effectively penetrate tissues saturated with it. Perhaps the single most important vitamin anyone can take, C is involved in more than 300 physiological functions that we know about, yet, unlike most other animals, we cannot make it for ourselves. It is extremely important for neutralizing toxins, and the body's demand for it soars in illness and in stress.

Dr Cathcart, who has treated some 9,000 patients with massive doses of vitamin C over the last ten years, has in some cases of severe candida overgrowth used from 15g up to an astounding 200g in patients extremely

Leon Chaitow: focus on the immune system

Naturopathic consultant Leon Chaitow, Senior Lecturer at Westminster University, and author of the UK's pioneering book on candida, *Candida Albicans*, believes that there is nothing prescription anti-fungals such as nystatin can do that natural anti-fungals cannot do better. He advocates using herbal anti-bacterial agents in combination with probiotics to focus on helping the immune system get back in charge. He says:

> One of the real problems with the superbugs is their interaction with other co-factors such as candida. An immune compromised person with candida who picks up one of the superbugs can find themselves with toxic shock or another condition called scalded skin syndrome.

The theory is that if the candida is dealt with and its output of immune-suppressive and metabolism-altering toxins is stopped, the immune system stands a better chance of throwing off other infections, even without antibiotics.

Probably the only naturopath currently working within Britain's National Health Service, Chaitow uses a herbal combination of the natural anti-viral and immune system helper echinacea with hydrastis (goldenseal) and berberis plants as a source of the anti-candida compound berberine, backed up with doses of Replete, a special probiotic bacterial supplement designed to help quickly recolonize the gut with helpful bacteria. He says:

> Probiotics have their own antibiotic effect as well as helping with the detoxification process. Natural treatments like these give us a much more hopeful prospect than doing nothing, which is where drug-based therapy is going to end up as the superbugs get stronger.

tolerant to ascorbic acid (the chemical name for vitamin C). You do not need to go that far. He advocates finding how much you need – and it varies all the time – by loading yourself with it until you start to feel loose. This test to bowel tolerance shows you that you are now saturated with vitamin C, and you can ease off. The cheapest way of taking large doses of vitamin C is in powder form. 'Raw' ascorbic acid may be too much for sensitive stomachs; if so, look for a buffered, ascorbate form. Vitamin C has been used to help cancer patients better tolerate chemotherapy, so it may be worth while combining it with prescription anti-fungals if you go that route.

The dreaded die-off reaction

With both prescription and natural anti-fungals there is one problem that has to be faced: the dreaded die-off reaction. Also known as the Herxheimer reaction, this is not a side-effect of the anti-fungals, but the result of toxins and wastes released as candida organisms are destroyed. When some of these anti-fungals work, they work quickly. The toxins have to be absorbed, neutralized and eliminated. While this job is carried out you may well feel tired and nauseous, and have headaches or what appears to be a worsening of your condition. This should be temporary, and you will be left feeling better than when you started. This reaction is a sure sign that candida is in your system and has been successfully targeted.

Because of the rapid increase in toxic load, it is important to support your liver with herbal or nutritional supplements while this is happening. The consensus opinion is that the die-off reaction, although welcome, can be minimized by gradually easing into the anti-candida regime. Start cutting out sugar while introducing probiotic supplements (*see below*) over the first two weeks. You can then begin reducing carbohydrates. When you introduce anti-fungals, start with small doses and build up. Some are produced in different strengths to make this easier to do.

Probiotics

This involves the use of supplements of the 'friendly' *Lactobacillus* and *Bifido* bacteria which live in the gut and stop candida from overgrowing but which are wiped out by antibiotic therapy.

This is a vital part of candida treatment and prevention. You must recolonize your intestines with beneficial bacteria, otherwise you will never bring candida permanently back into balance. The lactic acid bacteria normally dominant in a healthy gut also support your digestion and, some researchers believe, may also enhance the immune system.

Microbiologist Dr Nigel Plummer says:

> The normal flora of the gut are known to be important in preventing infections. But antibiotics can have a devastating effect on them, sometimes eliminating them completely. Probiotics may well play a very important role in re-establishing normal flora.

Tests have shown that when our 'friendly' bacteria are in place, it takes 1 milllion salmonella organisms to cause disease. When they are not there, it takes only ten.

Probiotics: the research evidence

Support for the use of Probiotics has finally come from the medical establishment with the publication of a review of the scientific literature conducted by researchers at the University of Washington, School of Medicine in Seattle and published in the *Journal of the American Medical Association* in 1996. They concluded:

> There is now evidence that administration of selected micro-organisms is beneficial in the prevention and treatment of certain intestinal and, possibly, vaginal, infections. In an effort to decrease the reliance on antimicrobials, the time has come to carefully explore the therapeutic applications of biotherapeutic agents.

Lactic acid bacteria in the small intestine in particular are associated with health benefits, but these are also the most vulnerable to antibiotics. Scientists at a British company developed Replete, a microbial replacement programme designed to be used for seven days after antibiotic treatment to repopulate the small intestine. Each dose of Replete provides 30 billion living organisms of three lactic acid bacteria: *Lactobacillus acidophilus*, *Bifido bacterium* and *Lactobacillus casei*, along with what are called prebiotics, substances needed for these bacteria to flourish.

Three different strains are used because they normally inhabit different regions of the small intestine; taken as a supplement they attach themselves to different areas of the wall of the intestine so that there is no spare ecological niche for candida to exploit. The prebiotics are high concentrations of the specific fructo-oligosaccharides, naturally-occurring types of sugars found in plants, that are preferred by lactic acid bacteria but cannot be used by disease-producing organisms.

Replete is a relatively expensive, short-term, supplement aimed at intensively reseeding the small intestine. Many practitioners recommend it at the start of an anti-candida treatment. Treatment should then be continued with normal probiotic products – daily supplements of *acidophilus*, the most important bacteria in the small intestine, and also of *bifido* bacteria, which will re-establish the balance in the large intestine.

Be warned that not all probiotic supplements are worth taking. Some contain very few viable bacteria, not matter what their labels may claim. Many manufacturers seem to have missed the point that they are dealing with live organisms which are fragile outside their normal environment and do not survive, in large numbers, the standard techniques used to produce and store vitamin and mineral pills and capsules. They must be freeze-dried early in the process or they will be unstable. The bacteria are also fussy about the company they keep,

Case study: Anne

Anne, 34, is Press Officer for a national charity. She says she has '95 per cent beaten off candida' using diet and supplements and changing the pace and style of her life.

She first started feeling ill about five years ago when she was living in London. She had flu-like symptoms and mouth ulcers, and felt run down. Then she moved to Somerset to start a new job and within nine months went down with a viral infection from which she never really recovered.

She was diagnosed as having an allergy to dairy foods, so cut them out of her diet. Within about four months, 'I virtually had ME (post-viral fatigue syndrome) without having ME – I was extremely paralysed with tiredness. I went to work because I had to, then I would struggle home and lie on the sofa all night. I had a lot of aching pains in my joints and was quite foggy in my brain. It felt like instead of having blood coursing through my veins I had cotton wool. It was terrifying, because I didn't know what was wrong with me.'

After four months she was diagnosed as having candida, 'and it all fell into place – all the symptoms I had.'

Her nutritional therapist started her on Replete, the short-term intensive bacterial supplement that helps to repopulate the gut with friendly bacteria, put her on an anti-candida diet and recommended supplements. In addition to the no-sugar, no-yeast, no-alcohol regime Anne was also avoiding dairy foods and a few others because of allergies, and she gave up coffee. 'Within six weeks I began to feel better, and I got better and better. I had been slightly over-weight, which hadn't helped matters and the weight started to fall off – I have lost 3 stone now!'

She is still sticking fairly closely to the diet. She still does not drink, she avoids bread because of the yeast content (eating yeast-free rye bread or crispbreads instead), and virtually the only fruit she has is an odd banana. She does have sweets now and then, and the occasional biscuit. She reintroduced vinegar, banned because of its yeast and mould content, then dropped it again because it seemed to provoke her old symptoms. 'I'm a little easier on the diet than when I was really ill,' she says. 'I've been on the anti-candida diet for virtually two years and I can't really see a day when I will go back to a sugary, yeasty diet and drink alcohol. I'm on this diet for life, and I'll keep taking supplements to look after my immune system. The thing is it's a healthy diet; it doesn't do you any harm to be on an anti-candida diet and it keeps the weight off.'

She has cut down on the number of supplements she was taking. She now regularly takes an *acidophilus* supplement, evening primrose oil (which she finds helps with premenstrual tension), vitamin C and calcium to balance the fact that she does not eat dairy products. She takes a one-week course of Replete if she feels particularly tired for no good reason or starts to feel achy.

'Occasionally, if I overdo it, it feels as if my immune system stops working properly, then I go down with bugs and viruses, get ill for a few days or feel exhausted. But I'm beginning to think everyone gets like that now and then; it's probably nothing to do with candida any more.'

She thinks her problems stemmed from the poor diet she was eating while she was living in London. It was basically a single working woman's diet, and she says: 'I never cooked. I either ate out or warmed up convenience food. I had sweet sticky drinks, ate loads of rubbish.' On top of that she had been on the contraceptive pill for years, another risk factor for candida, and then went through a period of severe stress, moving out of London to a new job in a new place where she had no friends and going back to live with her parents.

To improve her health she has done much more than go on a diet and take supplements. She started seeing a counsellor to deal with the feelings she experienced of being severely debilitated but having no support or understanding from the people around her. She started having regular massage, took up yoga and did a course in the Alexander Technique, a system of postural re-education that enables people to move with more relaxation and poise. 'I changed my lifestyle and learned to pace myself more,' she says. 'I am much, much fitter. I don't get all the aches I used to have, that were so bad I thought I had arthritis in my hands. I will never forget that feeling of utter fatigue I used to have. "Fatigue" doesn't describe it. It's driving home and then sitting in the car thinking, "Am I going to be able to walk up the garden path?" '

and mixing them with fillers or herbs – or even with other 'helper' bacteria – does not always work. Moreover, unless the bacteria used are of the right strain – the best are human strain – they will not survive in large numbers when introduced into the digestive system. Finally, probiotic bacteria need to be protected from moisture, heat and light and should be stored, whether in the shop or at home, in the refrigerator.

The effects of supplementation with the right sort of probiotic can sometimes be dramatic, even without the diet and anti-fungal agents. Studies by Harvard scientists at Boston City Hospital and published in the *Lancet*, for example, showed that when alcoholics with severe liver problems were given *Lactobacillus acidophilus* supplements, their clinical status and mental confusion significantly improved.

Yoghurt is a food which helps to put good bacteria back into the gut. However, not all types of yoghurt are able to do this. When I was editor of *Here's Health* magazine I surveyed every yoghurt manufacturer, asking them to tell us what organisms they used in their yoghurt. Quite a few would not say. Some were using organisms not far removed from slime moulds. Only a handful were using *acidophilus* and *bifido* bacteria in meaningful amounts.

On the plus side, a six-month study published in the *Annals of Internal Medicine* showed that women with recurrent candida infections had three times fewer infections if they consumed yoghurt containing *Lactobacillus acidophilus* every day. It also seems to be effective against immediate symptoms when applied direct to the vagina. The message is that yoghurt may help but will not cure. To recolonize the gut you need billions of the right sort of active bacteria and supplements are the way to get them. Look on yoghurt as an optional extra, if dairy foods suit you, and make sure it is a natural live variety, with no added sugar.

The argument for yoghurt is that it is supposedly easier to digest than milk and cheese. However, remember that dairy foods of whatever type are another relatively recent addition to our diet and many people cannot tolerate them at all. There is also the problem that lactose, the sugar in milk, feeds candida. The irony here is that our normal, helpful residents, *Lactobacillus acidophilus*, produce lactase, the enzyme that digests lactose.

Healing the gut

The final part of the anti-Candida protocol involves healing the damage Candida has done to your gut. You will also need to start correcting any slight nutritional deficiencies you may have and take steps to restore the efficiency of your digestion so that these do not reoccur. Many of these nutrients will also have positive effects on your immune system, which will then enable your natural defences to recover from being temporarily overwhelmed by candida and its side-effects.

By following the dietary recommendations above, you will already have eliminated many of the foods that could be contributing to the problem by aggravating the damage to your gut. There are specific nutritional and botanical supplements that can help to heal the damage, reduce inflammation, correct nutritional deficiencies and restore your metabolic balance and digestive efficiency. Those marked with a star are highly recommended.

- **Glutamine***. This amino acid is the primary nutrient for the cells of the intestine, the main nutrient needed for intestinal repair and the primary energy source of the immune system. The cells of the gastrointestinal tract are fast-growing, and until the 1970s it was thought that, like most others, they ran on glucose. Then researchers from the National Institutes of Mental Health in the USA discovered that it was glutamine which fed them. During illness and stress the body's requirement for glutamine soars to levels that are unlikely to be provided in the diet and it is so important that the body will break down muscle tissue to get it.

According to Dr Douglas Wilmore of Harvard Medical School, 'There is so little glutamine in food that barely enough is available even when we are healthy' (quoted in *Glutamine, The Ultimate Nutrient* by Judy Shabert and Nancy Ehrlich, Avery, 1994). At least three separate hospital studies (at Harvard, and in Germany and Sweden) have shown that the muscle-wasting which seems to be inevitable in patients undergoing major surgery can be alleviated by adding glutamine to their nutrition drips. Insufficient gluta-mine is thought to be a major factor in the development of leaky gut and, as if all that were not enough, it has been used, again in hospitals, to help the liver cope with massive toxic overload. Involved in the production of powerful anti-oxidants, gluta-mine is the liver's main protective chemical.

We do manufacture glutamine in the body from other amino acids, so officially it is not an essential amino acid, meaning that, we do not need to have it in our diets. However, unofficially, authorities such as nutritional biochemist Dr Jeff Bland have upgraded glutamine to 'essential non-essential' status. This means that if you want the best chance of healing a leaky gut and recovering, in general, from candida, you will benefit from taking a regular glutamine sup-plement. The cheapest way of doing this is to take it in powder form (as l-glutamine).

- **Fructo-oligosaccharides** (FOS). These may be con-tained in your probiotic supplement, as they provide *Bifido* bacteria in particular with the growth factors they need so that, among other things they can produce butyric acid (*see below*).

- **Butyric acid***. This is another preferred food source for the cells in the intestine. A supplement (as serine butyrate or calcium or magnesium butyrate) may help encourage the process. Be warned, however: butyric acid in powder form smells like vomit (in fact it is what gives vomit its aroma)!
- **N acetyl glucosamine (NAG)**. This forms an integral part of the collagen 'glue' that holds together the mucous membranes lining the intestines.
- **Magnesium and vitamin C**. Magnesium, which is important for the health of mucosal cells and vitamin C, which is vital for healing mucosal membranes and connective tissue, are often supplemented together as magnesium ascorbate, a stomach-friendly buffered form of vitamin C, which also helps support the immune system and the stress glands, the adrenals.
- **Vitamin A**. Essential for healing tissues lining the gut, vitamin A is best taken as beta-carotene, which the body then uses to make as much vitamin A as it needs with no toxicity problems. Carotenes have been found to be low in candida sufferers.
- **Essential fatty acids.** Toxins produced by candida, alcohol and an imbalance in the carbohydrate and protein ratio in your diet interfere with one of the body's most important biological catalysts, an enzyme that controls the production of a special family of chemical messengers known as eicosanoids, whose best-known members are the prostaglandins. These hormone-like chemical messengers go everywhere and do everything, including switching on and off the inflammatory processes involved in allergies and damage to membranes in the gut. The most important thing to remember about eicosanoids is that they are produced in the body from essential fatty acids, raw materials that are as important to our health as vitamins and minerals. Essential fatty acids, like other

vital nutrients, have to be supplied in our diets; we get them from the fats in our food.

Most people have picked up the message that too much saturated fat is a 'bad thing'. However, we have now gone too far in the other direction and are packing our diet with highly processed polyunsaturated fats. We are not getting enough of the essential fatty acids we need, which belong to the omega-3 family and are only available in significant quantities in cold-pressed seed and nut oils and in certain types of fish. According to Harvard's Dr Donald Rudin, omega-3 levels are down 80 per cent compared to our diet 100 years ago. He has seen dramatic results in patients given supplements of the right type of oils, after setting up a 44-patient pilot study that confirmed his theory that 'a new kind of epidemic of modern malnutrition' is in progress.

To readjust the balance in favour of health, most practitioners agree that in dealing with candida, mega-supplements of essential fatty acids are necessary, and they need to be minimally processed. You can use cold-pressed extra virgin olive oil or fresh flax seed (linseed) oil, but you will probably be advised to take dietary supplements as well. These are usually a combination of oils to provide the broad-spectrum fatty acids you need, from sources such as flax seed, evening primrose, borage and fish oils. Flax seed is the richest source of omega-3s. The naturopathic physician Dr Michael Murray reviewed the evidence and found that more than 60 health conditions have been shown to respond to fatty-acid supplementation. He recommends taking a tablespoonful of cold-pressed flax seed oil a day.

Helping the immune system

Changing your diet and using the supplements described will automatically help your immune system rediscover an ability to deal with candida by removing many of the other anti-nutrients and toxins it has to deal with. Among these are potentially toxic chemicals naturally produced as a by-product of using oxygen, which are mopped up by an important class of nutrients known as anti-oxidants. Dietary change and supplementation will also help provide high-quality fuel and a direct tonic through, for example, the restoration of the correct balance of bacteria in the intestine. Other nutrients you can consider in a bid to help put your immune system back on top form include:

- *Eleutherococcus senticosus*. Known as Siberian ginseng, this herb in fact is not a ginseng at all, but has similarities in that it is what is known as an adaptogen, and helps the body adapt to stress. There is a massive amount of research to prove its helpful effects on the immune system, and it has been used on everyone from cosmonauts to factory workers and athletes. Trials show that it reduces infections and can boost recovery. In Britain it has become a staple nutrient for triathletes, for whom infections and injuries due to the stress of training and competing have previously been an occupational hazard.
- **Selenium**. This trace element is an important anti-oxidant, which research shows can improve immune system function. It is no longer present in our soil due to modern farming practices and is subsequently getter rarer in our food.
- **Zinc**. This is another anti-oxidant mineral that helps the immune system. Research suggests that many people with candida overgrowth are zinc-deficient.
- **Co-enzyme Q10**. Also known as ubiquinone, co-enzyme Q10 has become one of the most well-researched single nutrients of all time. Its impact on the prevention and treatment of heart disease has been mirrored by startling findings in breast cancer and immune system disorders. Scientifically established by

Water

'Hairy bags of water' that we are, as sports nutrition expert Dr Michael Colgan describes us, it is odd that we forget that 'The most important nutrient in your body is pure water'. We are 70–80 per cent water. 'The quality of your tissues, their performance, and their resistance to injury, is absolutely dependent on the quantity and quality of the water you drink,' says Dr Colgan.

Dr F Batmanghelidj, who discovered a water cure for peptic ulcers while imprisoned by revolutionary guards in his native Iran, goes even further. He contends that many diseases originate in chronic dehydration. As only 25 per cent of the body is solid matter, the water content of it may be more important than the rest of us. It is true that we generally do not get enough pure water, while most of our common beverages contain diuretic caffeine, which means that although they are thirst-quenching we end up with a net loss of fluid. It is important to adjust this, particularly when eliminating candida toxins. He says:

> Your body needs an absolute minimum of six to eight 8-ounce glasses of water a day. The best times to drink water (clinically observed in peptic ulcer disease) are: one glass one half-hour before taking food . . . and a similar amount two and one half hours after each meal.

Exercise

Regular exercise increases energy, improves circulation, increases the elimination of toxins through the lungs and skin, and it is vital for making sure the lymphatic system is in good working order. The lymphatic fluid contains surveillance and scavenging cells of the immune system, as well as being the route by which we absorb those all-important fatty acids. Unlike the blood, however, lymph does not have a dedicated pump to make sure it circulates. Instead, it relies on gravity and on the contraction of the muscles. So we need to get them moving!

Regular exercise will improve your strength and stamina without sacrificing suppleness. Brisk walking and light weight-training balanced with relaxation and stretching is an ideal starting programme. It is important not to follow the example of many athletes who should know better and stretch before you work out; never stretch when your body is cold. Before exercise, you should loosen up and warm up. After exercise, when your muscles are warm, is the time to stretch.

The advantage of a system of exercise such as yoga, is that classes and self-practice sessions are generally organized so that the most intense stretches come after moves which warn and warm the parts which are going to be worked hard. In addition, breathing techniques and 'locks', or specific muscular contractions, can be used to generate internal heat. Yoga, which has been tried and tested for thousands of years, can range from the most gentle to the extremely vigorous, and is the simplest, most complete and most beneficial form of exercise, which not only strengthens the body, but can also correct physical imbalances and improve your capacity to shift oxygen round your system. You may also like to investigate yoga therapy, which applies yoga techniques to help people with specific health problems. 'Yoga is a holistic system of exercise that strengthens and relaxes the body, creating more calm within us, physically, emotionally and mentally,' says London's Yoga Biomedical Trust.

Moulds and yeasts in the environment

If you are dealing with candida overgrowth, you may well find that you feel unwell if you are living or working with yeasts and moulds, even if you avoid them in your diet.

Check your home and workplace for damp, dark places where yeasts and moulds might flourish. They naturally occur in soil, air and water, so you will never eliminate them entirely, but it makes sense to avoid places where they may be particularly abundant. You may be surprised to find quite a few sources around you: indoor plants and flower pots, piles of leaves or compost, old books, old furniture, damp mattresses and bedding that has not been aired, damp basements, bathrooms and kitchens, and rooms where washing is left to dry.

In addition to the basic programme outlined in this chapter, there are a number of other factors to deal with, such as stress, which we will explore in the following chapters.

But is all this really necessary? The short answer is yes. There are other approaches to treatment, such as homoeopathy and traditional Chinese medicine, which are not as demanding for the patient. There are also specialized allergy treatments that have claimed some success. However, there is very little published research to guide anyone seeking effective treatment for chronic candida overgrowth, and the most promising-sounding clinical reports and anecdotal success stories are, in the main, based on variations on the basic protocol given here.

The anti-candida diet without anti-fungals will not be effective. In Germany, physicians now believe that if we just remove sugar and yeast the candida seems to be driven into the deeper layers of the intestinal walls, where it is even more difficult to eradicate. From an ecological point of view this makes sense: a starving population intensifies its search for food.

Leave out supplementation with probiotics and, as has been shown with antibiotics, the danger is that candida will bounce right back as soon as you stop the anti-fungals or slip up on your diet. And miss out the healing of your damaged intestinal walls and you may continue to suffer many of your original problems, particularly

inflammation and allergic-type responses. You may them
end up having to restrict your diet much more severely.

Your final supplement is the RRR prescription, a combination of three essential ingredients that are often
ignored even in the most well thought-out regimes.
Without them, however, you will not get better. They are
relaxation, rest and recuperation, and we will be looking
at the ways in which you can get them in the following
chapters.

CHAPTER 6

Natural therapies: an overview

So far we have looked at ways of tackling candida over-growth through nutrition. Healing the gut through the gut seems fair enough, as we have seen that a candida problem is primarily an ecological one, with disturbances in the habitat – your intestines – leading to imbalances in health. But the micro-ecology of the gut is also part of a larger environment – the whole body – and that is part of an even bigger system including, but not limited to, your mind, your emotions, your spirituality and, of course, the world and people around you. In the next chapters we will look at some of the holistic systems of healing that can be used alongside nutrition in the treatment of candida overgrowth.

A friend of my family describes himself as an 'ordinary' doctor. He says that all this holistic stuff is beyond him. Now retired, he doctored in the country community in which he still lives for more than 40 years. I have spoken to many of his old patients, who fondly remember the times he sorted out a housing problem, came up with a part-time job and encouraged what is still a flourishing social club for older people. He retained his good manners and charming bedside manner through many a horrendous week of being called out to deaths and sudden emergencies in the middle of the night. To him it was all part of being a human being, not being a doctor.

Nowadays, we would probably say he was practising holistic medicine – even though he was not averse to prescribing antibiotics – and it has to be said that it is a type of holistic medicine that is beyond most alternative and complementary therapists. So let us not get carried away with the idea that the only good medicine is non-orthodox, non-hospital-based medicine. Your doctor is just as capable of taking a true holistic view of your problem as a natural therapist. However, it is true to say that, most of the time, your doctor does not have the time to do so. In some conditions it may also not be very important – when you have a simple, once-only problem and you want help resolving it. But with candida things can get more complex, and it can be valuable to see a practitioner who is not going to just treat the symptoms, but attempt to find out what is really causing your problem.

As we have seen, when it comes to treating the symptoms of candida, you might be lucky with a single burst of anti-fungal medication and bounce back to health, but it is more likely that, even if the treatment manages to remove the symptoms, you will only enjoy a temporary respite. For that reason, a practitioner of alternative or complementary medicine may want to explore different areas of your life to find out how the elements in this big picture are contributing to your problem with candida.

For instance, they will want to assess your level of stress and establish how you are dealing with it. Stress affects your immune system and can lay you open to infections and other illnesses. So what is happening at work, at home, with your family, your friends, or in your love life may be important, as might what you do for relaxation. If it becomes obvious that you are worried about work, you are not sleeping well, you are missing meals and you are starting to get pains in your stomach then there is little point asking you to take on a massive and life-altering schedule of treatment involving a total change of diet and taking a large amount of pills at every meal-time – you're stressed enough already! Treatment can always be adapted to your personal situation – that is what holistic medicine is all about. The best treatment for you may be a holiday, combined with a realistic assessment of what, if anything, you can do about your situation.

On a more basic level, your eating habits may have a considerable part to play in your problem, and it may well help if you consult a nutritional therapist, a naturopathic physician or a doctor or natural health practitioner trained in nutrition. There are also a variety of other approaches that either address the candida problem from a totally different perspective, such as ayurveda, traditional Chinese medicine, herbal medicine and homoeopathy, or that may contribute in smaller ways to the big picture, such as chiropractic, osteopathy, shiatsu and other physical therapies. Most of these therapies would claim to be one or all of the following:

- holistic, aiming to treat the whole person, not just the symptoms
- complementary, meaning that they can be used in conjunction with orthodox medical treatment and may enhance its effectiveness; also that treatments should complement the natural ecology of the body, working with it, not against it
- alternative, offering a real alternative to conventional medicine; treatment may be adversely affected by mixing the two (antibiotics and probiotics, for example)
- natural, aiming to use remedies that are natural, rather than synthetic, based on the experience that these are better tolerated by the body, are generally less toxic, and work with the body rather than against it.

A fundamental principle of complementary and alternative therapies is the most basic naturopathic belief in the healing power of nature. This translates into a belief, common throughout most of the therapies, that the body heals itself, given the chance. Remedies, supplements and techniques do not heal, nor does the practitioner. The practitioner's job is to:

- treat the patient, not the disease
- help the patient remove the obstacles to healing (which could be biochemical, structural, psychological or social)
- make sure the raw materials are available (which may be in the form of diet, supplements, remedies or ener-getic-vibrational input)
- make sure the opportunity is given (through relax-ation, rest and recuperation, even if it is only in the hour or so a week of therapy) for the body's innate self-healing ability to operate.

Because of the honest attempt most complementary and alternative therapies make to address health prob-lems on several levels at once, it is difficult to make a distinction between whether they treat the mind or the body; however, many do have a particular focus; they fall very roughly into two main categories – physical and psychological therapies – with a possible third cate-gory of energy or vibrational therapies.

- **Physical therapies** are those which work obviously and directly on the body in a very physical way, both outside and in. Examples are chiropractic, osteopathy, massage, reflexology and other forms of bodywork, nutritional therapy, medical herbalism and colonic therapy.
- **Psychological therapies** aim to help the body by bene-fiting the mind and emotions. Examples are meditation teaching, psychotherapy, hypnotherapy, counselling, relaxation and biofeedback.
- **Energy or vibrational therapies** work on the principle that illness only appears in the physical body after an imbalance or interruption has occurred at a more subtle level, in the body's natural energy, vital force

or life force. Examples are acupuncture, homoeopathy, flower remedies and gem, crystal and colour healing.

Categories like this are not entirely satisfactory, and there are many therapies – such as shiatsu, for instance – which overlap the categories. They are also not broad enough to encompass ancient and modern natural therapies that are in fact complete systems of healing. Examples are:

- ayurveda, the 3,000-year-old traditional Indian system of medicine, which includes bodywork, herbs, diet, exercise and a spiritual component
- traditional Chinese medicine, also thousands of years old, which uses acupuncture, herbs, dietary advice, massage and both internal and external arts of energy manipulation
- naturopathic medicine, which traditionally focused on the basic principles of light, air, water and food, and in its modern, eclectic incarnation incorporates clinical nutrition, herbs, homoeopathic remedies, bodywork, hydrotherapy, therapeutic fasting and counselling and, like the ancient systems, emphasizes the possibility of building optimum health and preventing disease, rather than just treating it when it develops.

Despite these problems, however, the categories are useful in providing an overview of the therapies on offer, and the chapters that follow are based on them.

CHAPTER 7

Treating the body

Medical herbalism

The West's original holistic medical system has its roots in ancient Greece and its future in modern scientific exploration of the healing powers of plants. Although herbal remedies such as garlic and milk thistle have a place in the overall candida approach using diet and supplementation, a specialist practitioner of herbal medicine would probably regard this as a piecemeal, symptomatic use of herbs. While a modern herbalist would undoubtedly use specific anti-fungals and liver support, the overall aim is to nudge the body back into balance by bringing its weaker systems up to par and enhancing elimination and detoxification so that the immune system can do the job it is designed to do.

In addition to the herbal remedies already mentioned, another effective way of using plants is by taking the juice of organically grown herbs. In Germany, plant juices are widely used in this way; they are regarded as being more potent than teas and dried remedies. Many people juice their own medicinal plants every day, but there is a wide range of commercially produced juices. German pharmacist Walther Schoenenberger is widely credited with having discovered and set the standards for producing and bottling these powerful juices while retaining their full biological activity. His research started nearly 50 years ago. Two plant juices that are especially recommended as a combination for use in candida are ramsons (*Allium ursinum*) which Siegfried Gursche, author of a book on Schoenenberger called *Healing with Herbal Juices*, describes as 'a wild cousin of the garlic family', and wormwood (*Artemisia absinthium*), which in this form provides a high concentration of bitters.

Traditional Chinese medicine (TCM)

Combining the use of herbs, dietary recommendations and acupuncture, TCM diagnosis also looks at where the body is out of balance, but in a way that seems peculiar to many Western minds. It emphasizes that the body is in a constant state of change and treatment aims to restore a dynamic balance in the way it uses chi, a subtle energy that is channelled throughout the body in channels known as meridians. Acupuncture involves the practitioner placing extremely fine needles at specific points along these meridians. The needles pierce the skin, but it does not hurt, although there may be some soreness or a sensation of numbing as the point is treated. Indeed, acupuncture is routinely used in China to anaesthetize parts of the body for surgery.

A TCM diagnosis sounds bizarre to Western scientists, as a condition may be rather poetically described as being due to 'liver heat rising' or 'kidney yin deficiency'. That is because the practitioner is looking at the balance and interplay of the familiar Chinese Five Elements, which are like five different expressions or moods of the chi energy. The Elements are Wood (developing and generating), Fire (expanding and radiating), Earth (stabilizing and centering), Metal (solidifying and contracting) and Water (gathering and sinking). Each has a yin and yang aspect, or a soft–hard, negative–positive feeling. These Elements are associated with particular pairs of organs, which is again very different from Western medicine: the heart/small intestine (Fire), kidneys/bladder (Water), liver/gall bladder (Wood), lungs/large intestine (Metal) and pancreas/spleen/stomach (Earth).

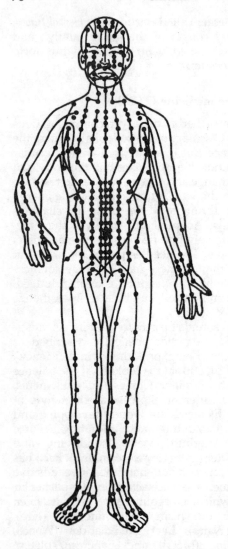

Fig. 4 The acupuncture energy meridians

To a TCM practitioner, this is not complicated or mysterious, simply another way of looking at the interplay of energy in the body. And the body gives all the clues the skilled practitioner needs to be able to read what is going on inside. First there are the symptoms, of course, but these are less important than how they are produced, as different people may manifest what looks like the same disease from a different combination of imbalances. So the TCM practitioner will take several pulses and carefully examine the tongue, also taking into account the colour and condition of the skin, hair, nails and so on to make a diagnosis.

Treatment is usually with a combination of herbs and acupuncture. Many practitioners use dried herbs, which you will be directed to cook up with boiling water into a foul-tasting soup – I have yet to meet anyone who found their herbal brew delicious! Several sessions of acupuncture are normally required.

It seems likely that acupuncture enables the TCM practitioner to influence the body's functioning directly through the nervous system, adding a dimension of treatment missing from other therapies.

Ayurveda

This is perhaps the oldest system of medicine in the world, and the dominant form of traditional medicine in India. Undeniably holistic, ayurveda contains everything from a way of matching your diet and remedies to your particular physiology, to techniques that address physical structural problems and the mental–emotional component of disease. It is becoming more available in the West from medical doctors who have taken further training, and is often offered in a simplified form using primarily herbal remedies and an adjustment to diet. Specific anti-candida remedies may be employed, but the emphasis is on enabling you to achieve a balance of the three *doshas* or energetic influences – *vatta, pitta* and *kapha* – in your system.

Osteopathy and chiropractic

At some point in your candida treatment, you will need to get the 'mechanics' of your body checked in case this is interfering with your recovery. Osteopaths and chiropractors specialize in manipulative techniques that aim to help you correct structural imbalances. Some of these may not be causing you any apparent problems, but a simple problem in the spine, for instance, can have far-reaching effects through the irritation of a nerve that may in turn cause an organ to become dysfunctional. This may be a direct knock-on effect involving a displaced vertebra mechanically pressing on a nerve alongside it, or a chronic muscular contraction causing a similar problem. It is also common for a structural problem, whether it is caused by stress leading to a chronic clenching of the muscles, by accidental trauma or just by bad postural habits, to cause tremendous muscular pressure on an internal organ.

A bodywork adage is that 'structure determines function'. This could translate into the idea that you are unlikely to be able to restore normal digestive function if you spend your days continually hunched over a desk, cramping your abdomen. As we have seen, your internal environment is not only sensitive to stress of all kinds, but is dependent on an efficient balance of acid and alkaline secretions, and on the ability of the gut to enjoy the freedom to move.

Hydrotherapy

Treatment with water can achieve some dramatic results. Hot and cold applications of water are a traditional naturopathic method that are being validated by modern research. You can boost your energy and your immune system by gradually building up your exposure to cold water so that after a period of around three months you can totally immerse yourself in cold water – and enjoy it! Research which followed the progress of people using this system of gradual exposure showed that the body adapts to the increasing immersion so that by the end of the three-month period, a soak in cold water feels like a perfectly normal way to start the day. Benefits in improved immune reponse were shown in fewer colds and infections and increased energy. The key is to start this process of 'hardening' very gradually, by first getting used to starting the day by soaking just your feet in cold water. Take your time and gradually get more of you under the water.

Bodywork

Different forms of bodywork are extremely valuable in candida. Partly this is due to the relaxation response they cause, enabling your body to begin to clear the toxic by-products of stress, which can result in an improvement in your immune system. Different forms of bodywork also claim to affect the body more deeply, either through reflex effects on nerves, trigger points and acupuncture points just under the surface of the skin, or by clearing, through manual pressure, any stagnated build-up of chemical toxins or energy blocks. These types of therapy include:

- **neuromuscular technique**, a sophisticated system of diagnosis and treatment which works on the soft tissue of the body, mainly with thumb pressure; it includes many different systems of treatment points on the body that can affect other tissues and organs through reflex action
- **massage**, which varies from types that are aimed purely at relaxation to a system that focuses on specific injuries or areas of muscular tension or tissue damage
- **shiatsu**, which operates on a meridian system, like

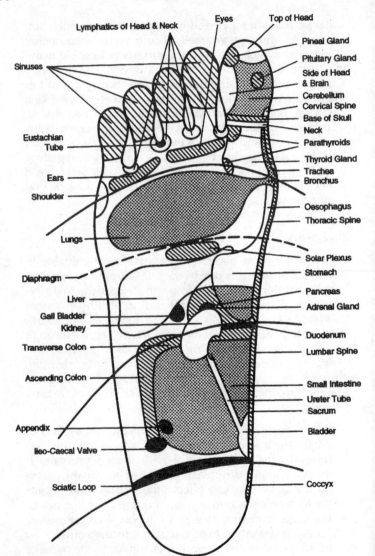

Fig. 5 Reflexology zones on the right foot

acupuncture, but with thumb, elbow, knee and hand pressure to points rather than needles, as well as the application of stretching and supportive holding techniques

- **reflexology**, which involves mainly thumb pressure and stroking to areas on the soles of the feet, on the basis that working on these areas affects organs and tissues of the body which are said to be connected to them through a system of reflexes

Aromatherapy

Aromatherapy combines the relaxing and stress-reducing benefits of massage with the bonus of the application of essential oils which can be aimed at specific disease conditions as well as at balancing your overall health. The oils work on many different levels, stimulating responses to their aroma in the brain, which can then produce profound changes in the body through the release of chemical messengers. They enter the bloodstream via the lungs and also, of course, through the skin, so that they can have an immediate local effect on tissues and organs. Some oils, such as tea tree, peppermint and eucalyptus oils, have anti-bacterial, anti-viral and anti-fungal activity; some, like lavender and bergamot, can help to produce a deep state of relaxation.

Colon hydrotherapy

A direct, mechanical way of giving your colon a clear-out, colonics are traditionally used as part of a detoxification programme to loosen faecal matter that may be impacted on the walls of the large intestine and to wash out harmful bacteria. As part of a treatment for candida overgrowth, the colon therapist can also take the opportunity to introduce 'helper' bacteria into the colon.

CHAPTER 8

Treating the mind and emotions

It is bad enough being barely able to get out of bed in the morning, worse still when you cannot think straight, and everything you eat either sends you back to sleep or gives you pain and bloating. It becomes even worse when your friends and loved ones eventually lose patience with your constant quest to find out what is wrong with you and start telling you to pull yourself together and join a gym or take a degree or go on holiday. Candida is not an illness that wins you friends and sympathy. You probably look perfectly normal, for one thing.

To make matters even worse, some of the toxins produced by candida can cross the blood-brain barrier, so, added to your general fatigue, you may well experience feelings of confusion, anxiety, depression (*see box*) or just not be able to think straight some of the time.

Depression

Depression can be dangerous, so see your primary care doctor if you experience symptoms including:

- mood swings
- early morning wakening
- low self-esteem
- unexplained pain or fatigue

This is the sort of state in which many people attempt to treat themselves for candida overgrowth. But how can you expect to make rational decisions about treatment? In truth, many people do not. So they switch from one new supplement to another, from one therapy to another, getting a bit better, then relapsing.

The answer to all this is: get support. Even if you are seeing a practitioner, get support as well. Contact a candida support group (see 'Useful addresses') or team up with a fellow sufferer you know. You might also consider counselling.

Counselling

Counselling can have immediate benefits. First, you will have somebody who is always there for you and always on your side. Secondly, you will have someone 'keeping score'. It can be easy to miss signs of improvement: symptoms that do not bother you any more. This can be just what you need to keep going when things get tough.

Thirdly, you will have someone with whom you can explore the internal processes associated with your illness and provides answers to the questions why me, why this, why now? You can take an objective look at what you expect from your family and friends. Many families actively resist someone going on a 'funny' diet and sabotage decisions to stay off chocolate or alcohol. Moreover, you can explore what life will be like when you are well. Will it mean you have more energy? Will that mean you will finally be able to do those things you've always wanted to do? And does that scare your family or your partner? Does it scare *you*? Bear in mind that you may have been ill for quite some time. Friends and family get used to you like that, and most people do not like change – and look suspiciously even at supposedly positive change.

Exploring the symbology of candida

Underlying all that, there are choices and experiences that have led you to the point at which you have candida. What is the deeper meaning behind it all? Many people find it helpful to explore the symbology of their illness. There is a school of thought that suggests that illness is an opportunity created to help you learn something. We are familiar with the fact that our 'other-than-conscious' mind may communicate with us through dreams, and that the language it uses is that of symbols. Similarly, your symptoms can be seen as an attempt to communicate what it is you need to learn. According to spiritual psychologist Thorwald Dethlefsen and his colleague Dr Rüdiger Dahlke, the authors of *The Healing Power of Illness*, the small intestine is often the location for fears about our survival, and is the place of processing and splitting, or analysis. Psychologically and physiologically, the digestive system 'has a mind of its own'. We have 'gut feelings' about things. The large intestine, where digestion is over but the residual water and nutrients are extracted, is to do with greed and the unconscious. Infection is seen as a 'conflict made flesh'. So in this language, candida overgrowth may be seen as a clear sign that something is eating away at you, something that may be getting out of control. According to Buddhist teacher Debbie Shapiro, it also implies that your normal environment is unbalanced or upset, maybe allowing unwanted energies or influences to enter your life.

Louise Hay, one of the world's leading interpreters of this other language, and author of *You Can Heal Your Life*, suggests that in candida a contributory factor may be a sustained pattern of thought that may include 'feeling very scattered, lots of frustration and anger'. She suggests the use of the affirmation: 'I give myself permission to be all that I can be, and I deserve the very best in life. I love and appreciate myself and others.'

Dealing with stress

On a more scientific basis, the fact that the entire gastro-intestinal tract is acutely affected by mental and emotional stress is widely accepted. Research by Dr Candace Pert and colleagues at the Brain Biochemistry Division of the USA's National Institutes of Mental Health, suggests the brain, glands, immune system and emotions may be linked by chemicals called neuropeptides, which include chemical messengers such as hormones and the not so well-known gut peptides. A leading researcher into mind–body links, Dr Ernest Rossi, says that the nerve and chemical communication system in the digestive organs is of the same order of complexity as the network of nerves in the spinal cord. This may begin to explain why working things out in your mind and emotions can be an important part of healing your candida. It is possibly why various forms of hypnotherapy are often successful in dealing with digestive disorders.

This also points up the urgent need to deal with stress. There is nothing wrong with a certain amount of stress. However the stress of life events that we feel powerless to control, or that goes on too long, takes us past the point where we feel enlivened, energized and excited and on to exhaustion. This level of stress depletes our reserves and suppresses our immune systems. Studies on students taking exams and on business executives have demonstrated how stress can lead to illness. However, it does not do so in everybody. A landmark study of 200 executives at Illinois Bell Telephone Company in the 1970s showed that only half of them reported serious illness, although all were subjected to much the same level of stress. Ian McDermott and Joseph O'Connor, trainers and consultants in neuro-linguistic programming (NLP), a system of modelling and teaching effective mental and physical skills, say:

The executives who stayed healthy had a different way of

thinking about events. They considered change to be an inevitable part of life and an opportunity to grow, not a threat to what they had achieved. They believed that while they could not always control what happened, they could control the impact of the problem.

McDermott and O'Connor believe that NLP techniques allow people to learn to give themselves more choices about how they respond to stress.

One of the ways to do this is by making sure that we believe positive things about ourselves. 'A belief in your own ability to control events in your life will automatically reduce the stress you suffer,' they say. Researchers at Stanford University have studied this mental set-up, which they call 'self-efficacy' They found that the more people believe they can cope with challenge, the less stress takes a toll of their bodies. People with this belief have stronger immune systems. McDermott and O'Connor's book *NLP and Health* is packed with suggestions and practical, effective exercises that can help you change unhelpful patterns of thinking and behaviour. And as the authors say, 'Choice comes from your control over your internal world, not the external world, which is neither predictable nor controllable.'

Traditional ways of regaining control of your inner world revolve around experiencing a sense of inner peace and harmony, enabling you to get things in perspective. Meditation and yoga, which in the classical tradition is actually the physical preparation for deep relaxation and meditation, are two ways of doing this. Transcendental Meditation (TM), one of the best-known systems of meditation, has been heavily researched by doctors and scientists, and has shown amazing health benefits from regular practice. The internal martial arts of t'ai chi and chi kung bring you to this experience of relaxation, peace and a sense of inner power through flowing movements or static postures in which you learn to experience the flow of your internal energy.

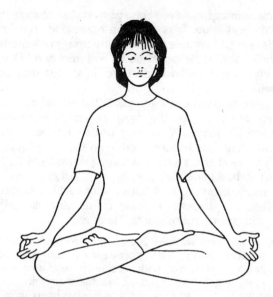

Fig. 6 The Lotus position

Gentle bodywork where static, non-invasive touch and holding is used, in contrast to deep, tissue work, may also enable you to experience this sense of relaxation and calm. Naturopath and osteopath Leon Chaitow calls these techniques 'stillpoint' therapies and has compared them to fasting, where nothing is being done to the body – it is simply being allowed to experience physiological rest.

In many of these non-activities, the mind may be active at some points. In visualizing yourself in total health, for instance, you need to be able to direct your thoughts consciously until you have a clear picture of yourself. In NLP techniques, you are encouraged to build a thorough mind-experience for yourself, preferably in full colour, and including sounds, smells and sensations. As we all know from having cried or cringed at a film or TV programme, images have the power to change our physiological state. It is as if the brain does not know what is real and what is not. So if you imagine something vividly enough, the brain–body will respond. Does it not make sense to have positive, healthful images of yourself?

In contrast, passive awareness is the key to autogenic training (AT), one of the most powerful methods of dealing with stress. A leading British teacher, Dr Kai Kermani, who has written a book on the technique, has used it to good effect even in what he terms 'catastrophic illness': it has benefited people with AIDS as well as many more common conditions such as arthritis, eczema and digestive diseases such as colitis, and is used in sport, education and business. He says:

> Most of our lives we have been taught to concentrate hard and actively. Usually our concentration is aim- and result-orientated . . . However, with passive concentration we are not trying to get there or indeed to achieve anything, all we are trying to do is sit back and watch what happens to our bodies and minds when we go through the AT training formulae [phrases] and instructions.

The AT instructions such as 'My right arm is heavy. My right arm is warm' are repeated in a set sequence until feelings of warmth and heaviness happen. Your heartbeat and breathing are slowed and calmed with similar instructions, which are built up in sequences until your body and mind can be conditioned to respond with total relaxation to a simple suggestion. Then AT can be used regularly to break the normal anxiety-ridden response to stress, a response that can disable the immune system, and replace it with a natural state of relaxed awareness. This allows the natural healing forces of the body to begin to work. As Dr Kermani says:

> This is why AT is so different from anything else. We think that we know at a conscious level what is best for us. In fact, it is the inner wisdom of our bodies and minds that

knows best, and if we allow them to communicate freely and without interference, they do their best for us.

Whichever way you choose to help your healing through your mind, what is important is to be able to experience, at least once, what it feels like to be deeply relaxed and unconcerned. Having been there, you then have a state to refer to and will find it easier to re-enter it.

CHAPTER 9

Life force and experimental therapies

Homoeopathy

This 200-year-old system developed by Dr Samuel Hahnemann uses highly diluted and energized or 'potentized' remedies that seem to be able to stimulate the body to heal itself. Homoeopathic treatment is based on the principle that 'like cures like', but also on obtaining a total picture of your symptoms.

The remedy that is exactly right for you may only emerge after hours of questioning and thought. Although homoeopathy acknowledges some 'specific' remedies that may be able to help most cases of a particular condition, such as outbreaks of flu and other epidemic illnesses, it is usually the case that ten people with candida overgrowth will each receive a different remedy.

Homoeopathy also claims to be the only system of medicine that has a way of identifying and clearing inherited predispositions to disease. It is another system that treats the whole person, not just the physical body.

Hahnemann not only showed that treating like with like is extremely effective, but introduced the idea of using extremely diluted doses of medicine which could be 'potentized' during preparation. Homoeopathy's success rate seemed to validate another of Hahnemann's major theories: he maintained that people's recovery from illness was often hampered because in their systems were 'miasms', inherited or acquired predispositions to disease that were operating on an energetic or vibrational level, not on the purely physical.

Homoeopathic medicine has some powerful assistance to give to the rebalancing of the bowel flora thanks to the breakthrough work done between 1910 and 1920 by Dr Edward Bach, a physician at University College Hospital, London, who later became pathologist and bacteriologist at the London Homoeopathic Hospital. Bach connected 'miasms' with his discovery that bacteria in the intestines were producing poisons and stopping people getting better. He introduced new remedies, which became known as Bach Bowel Nosodes, whose effects were to cleanse the entire intestinal tract. There are many organisms that live in the bowel, but Bach was able to classify them into seven different types. In time, he was able to predict which of the seven was causing a person's health problems simply by looking at their symptoms.

Bach's research was published in the medical journals of the time, and other physicians took on the future development of nosodes. Nosodes are sometimes prepared from a person's own bacteria and have been used in AIDS with apparently good results. This and the general homoeopathic approach are well worth considering in candida. First, homoeopathy claims to be able to reach the parts other systems of medicine cannot, clearing out inherited or acquired taints that could block the healing process. Also, as Drs Sheila and Robin Gibson of the Glasgow Homoeopathic Hospital have pointed out, 'Bach also found that certain homoeopathic remedies could change the bacterial flora of patients although no conventional drugs or dietary regimes had produced any significant change' (quoted in *Homoeopathy for Everyone*, Arkana, 1991). Clearly this research needs to be followed up by present-day bacteriologists.

Many homoeopathic practitioners today are still reluctant to use anything except homoeopathy. Bach, of course, was operating in an era before the advent of probiotic supplements made it relatively easy to make dramatic changes in intestinal bacterial counts. Nosodes remain as one option in homoeopathic treatment, with or without additional help from diet or probiotic supplements.

But Dr Bach did not stop there. He went on to develop flower remedies, which are widely available and easy to self-administer. The remedies are a collection of some 38 essences classified by the seven major psychological states that they aim to help. Dr Bach continued to look for more and more subtle ways of using remedies; he saw that patients' character traits and mental symptoms seemed to match the type of bacteria causing the problem, and he retired from practising medicine and devoted the rest of his life to a spiritual search, finding gentle flower remedies that could be prescribed on that basis, without the need for laboratory tests.

Building on the Bach tradition, many other countries have now developed their own essences. They include flower and gem essences from California and from the Australian bush. Their mechanism of action is unknown. Dr Richard Gerber suggests:

> Vibrational medicines such as flower essences, gem elixirs and homoeopathic remedies . . . utilize the energetic storage properties of water to transfer a frequency-specific, infor-mation-bearing quantum of subtle energy to the patient in order to effect healing at various levels of human func-tioning.

This is entirely speculative, however, and there are years of research ahead before it is established what is going on at this 'energetic' level of healing.

Geopathic stress and feng shui

Treating the root cause of your illness may involve you in moving house – or at least your bed. If you are sleeping in the wrong place you may be subjecting your-self to long-term input of harmful electromagnetic radiation. Geopathic stress is the description for disrup-tive energy which may be due to sources as varied as underground streams, ley lines or the intersection of lines of electromagnetic radiation known as Hartmann lines, which are thought to be laid out in a grid system all over the earth and are something to do with the planet's own electromagnetic field. Professional dowsers can nor-mally detect geopathic stress and there are many different ways of treating it if moving is out of the ques-tion, including shielding for your bed and plug-in devices.

Dealing with much the same problem from a totally different perspective is the ancient Oriental system of feng shui, or the art of placement. Feng shui masters are routinely consulted in the East to advise on how to improve the flow of energy in homes and businesses to ensure health and prosperity. Like geopathic stress, a house or office in the wrong place or with the wrong layout, dooms its occupants to the effects of sick building syndrome.

CHAPTER 10

How to find and choose a natural therapist

Finding a practitioner should not be too difficult. There are plenty of them around these days, and many are well trained and registered with professional associations that keep an eye on them. There has recently been an explosion of public interest in the natural therapies and a vast increase in the numbers of practitioners using them. A 1993 *New England Journal of Medicine* report estimated that people in the US are spending around $15 billion a year on this form of healing. In Australia, according to 1996 figures published in the *Lancet*, another mainstream medical journal, the figure is A$1 billion – Australians are estimated to be spending twice as much on alternative medicine as they do on pharmaceutical drugs.

Choosing the right practitioner is not so easy. You need to know that they can deal with your problem, and it is also important that you find them easy to get on with. In every therapy there are different approaches and different personalities. It is important to have a counsellor or practitioner who suits you. Many people feel that they are stuck with their first choice, and if things do not work out, it is their own fault. This is not true; you should shop around.

The best way to find a practitioner is through personal recommendation. Ask around. Your local health food store or alternative bookshop may be able to recommend someone. And if your doctor is sympathetic to complementary therapies, he or she will probably have an unofficial list of reliable local practitioners. Failing that, you will have to check on them yourself. You can tell a lot from a phone call, and even more from a visit to the clinic. Ask plenty of questions and use your intuition as well.

Here are some questions to ask:

- Where and when were you trained?
- How long was the course?
- Was that full or part time?
- What diplomas do you hold?
- Do you hold any other qualifications?
- How long have you been in practice?
- How long have you been in practice in this area?
- Where else have you practised?
- What methods of treatment do you use?
- What do they entail?
- Can you give an estimate of how many consultations I will need?
- How much does treatment cost?
- Have you successfully treated people for my condition?
- Do you have any testimonial letters I can look at, or would you mind if I contacted a previous patient of yours to find out exactly what the treatment involved?
- Are you a member of any professional association?
- Are you willing to work in conjunction with the treatment I am getting from my regular doctor or with another practitioner?

What is it like seeing a natural therapist?

Since most natural therapists, even in those countries with state health systems, still work privately, there is no established common pattern.

Although they may all share more or less a belief in the principles outlined in chapter 6, you are liable to come across individuals from all walks of life. You will find as much variety in dress, thinking and behaviour as there are fashions, ranging from the formal and sophisticated to the absolutely informal.

Equally, you will find their premises very different. Some will present a 'brass plaque' image, working in a clinic with a receptionist and brisk efficiency, while others will see you in their living room surrounded by plants and domestic clutter.

Remember, though, that while image may be some indication of status, it is little guarantee of ability. You are as likely to find a therapist of quality working from home as in a formal clinic.

Some characteristics, however, and probably the most important ones, are common to all natural therapists:

- They will give you far more time than you are used to with a family doctor. An initial consultation will rarely last less than an hour, and is often longer. They will ask you all about yourself so they can form a proper understanding of what makes you tick and what may be the fundamental cause(s) of your problem.
- You will have to pay for any remedies they prescribe, and they may well sell you these from their own stocks. They will also charge you for their time – though many therapists offer reduced fees for deserving cases or for people who genuinely cannot afford the full fee.

Sensible precautions

- Be sceptical of anyone who 'guarantees' you a cure. No one (not even doctors) can do that.
- Query any attempt to book you in for a course of treatment. Your response to any natural therapy is highly individual. Of course, if the practice is a busy one, booking ahead for one or two sessions might be

sensible. You should be able to cancel without penalty any sessions which prove unnecessary (but remember to give at least 24 hours' notice: some practitioners will charge you if you don't give enough notice).

- No ethical therapist will ask for fees in advance of treatment unless for special tests or medicines – and even this is unusual. If you are asked for 'down payments' of any sort, ask exactly what they are for. If you don't like the reasons, don't pay.

- Be wary if you are not asked about your existing medication and try to give precise answers when you are asked. Be especially wary if the therapist tells you to stop or change any medically prescribed drug without talking to your doctor first. (A responsible doctor should also be happy to discuss you and your medication with a therapist.)

- Note the quality of the therapist's touch if you choose any of the relaxation or manipulation techniques such as massage, aromatherapy or osteopathy. It should never be lingering or suggestive. If, for any reason, the therapist wants to touch you on the breasts or genitals, your permission should be sought first.

- If the practitioner is of the opposite sex you are entitled to have someone of your choice in the room at the same time. Be immediately suspicious if this is not allowed. Ethical therapists will not refuse this sort of request, and if they do, it is probably best to have nothing more to do with them.

What to do if things go wrong

A practitioner is in a position of trust, and is charged with a duty of care to you at all times. It does not mean you are 'entitled' to a 'cure' just because you've paid for treatment, but if you feel you are being treated unfairly, incompetently or unethically, you have several options:

- Tackle the matter at the source of the problem, with your practitioner, either verbally or in writing.
- If he or she works in a place such as a clinic, health farm or sports centre, tell the management. They also have a duty to protect the public and should treat complaints seriously and discreetly.
- Contact the practitioner's professional organization. It should have an independent panel that investigates complaints fully and disciplines its members.
- If the offence committed is a criminal one report it to the police (but be prepared for the problem of proving one person's word against another's).
- If you feel compensation is due see a lawyer for advice.

Short of a public court case, the worst thing for a truly incompetent or unethical practitioner is bad publicity. Tell everyone about your experiences. People only need to hear the same sort of comments from a few different sources and the practitioner will probably sink without trace. Before you do so, though, try the other measures first and give yourself time to consider things calmly. Vengeance is not very healing.

A word of warning Don't make malicious allegations without good reason. Such actions are themselves a criminal offence in most countries and you could end up in more trouble than the practitioner.

Summary

The reality is that there are few real crooks or charlatans in natural therapy. Despite the myth, there is little real money in it unless the therapist is very busy – and the chances are high that a busy therapist is a good one. Remember that no one can know everything and no specialist qualified in any field has to get 100 per cent in the exams to be able to practise. Perfection is an ideal, not a reality, and to err is human.

It is very much for this reason that taking control of your own health is perhaps the single most important lesson underlying this book. Taking control means taking responsibility for the choices you make, and this is one of the most significant factors in successful treatment.

No one but you can decide on a practitioner and no one but you can determine if that practitioner is any good or not. You will know this very easily, and probably very quickly, by the way you feel about the person and the therapy, and by whether or not you get any better.

If you are not happy, the decision is yours whether to stay or move on – and continue moving until you find the right therapist for you. Don't despair if you don't find the right person first time. There is almost bound to be the right person for you somewhere and your determination to get well is the best resource you have for finding that person.

Above all, bear in mind that many people who have taken this route before you have not only been helped beyond their most optimistic dreams, but have also found a close and trusted helper who will assist in times of trouble – and who may even become a friend for life.

APPENDIX A

Useful organizations

This listing is for information only and does not imply any endorsement, nor do the organizations listed necessarily agree with the views expressed in this book.

AUSTRALASIA

Australian Natural Therapists Association
PO Box 308
Melrose Park
South Australia 5039.
Tel 8297 9533
Fax 8297 0003

Australian Traditional Medicine Society
PO Box 442 or Suite 3, First Floor,
120 Blaxland Road
Ryde
NSW 2112
Tel 2808 2825
Fax 2809 7570

New Zealand Natural Health Practitioners Accreditation Board
PO Box 37–491
Auckland
Tel 9 625 9966

NORTH AMERICA

American Association of Naturopathic Physicians
PO Box 20386
Seattle
WA 98102
Tel 206 323 7610
Fax 206 323 7612

American Holistic Medical Association
4101 Lake Boone Trail, Suite 201
Raleigh
NC 27607
Tel 919 787 5146
Fax 919 787 4916

Canadian Holistic Medical Association
700 Bay Street
PO Box 101, Suite 604
Toronto
Ontario M5G 1Z6
Tel 416 599 0447

Diagnos-Techs
620 South 192nd Pl
#J-104
Kent
WA 98032
(1–800–87–TESTS)
For information about testing.

Great Smokies Diagnostic Laboratory
18a Regent Park Blvd
Asheville
NC 28806
Tel 1 800 522 4762
For information about testing

International Foundation for Homeopathy
PO Box 7
Edmonds
WA 98020
Tel 425 776 4147
Fax 425 776 1499

International Health Foundation
PO Box 3494
Jackson
TN 38303
Tel 901 427 8100
Fax 901 423 5402
The Foundation will provide a list of doctors in the USA and Canada who are interested in yeast-related illnesses.

Dr Robert F Cathbert MD
127 Second Street
Los Altos
California 94022
Tel 415 949 2822

Meridian Valley Clinical Laboratory
24030 132nd Ave SE
Kent
WA 98042
Tel 206 859 8700
For information about testing.

Phoenix Rising Yoga Therapy
PO Box 819
Housatonic
MA 01236

SOUTHERN AFRICA

South African Homoeopaths, Chiropractors and Allied Professions Board
PO Box 17055
0027 Groenkloof
S Africa
Tel 2712 466 455

UNITED KINGDOM

Action for ME
PO Box 1302
Wells BAS 1YE
Web site: http://www.afme.org.uk

British Acupuncture Council
Park House
206–208 Latimer Road
London W10 6RE
Tel 0181 964 0222

British Association for Autogenic Training and Therapy
6 Avenue Road
Malvern
Worcs WR14 3AG

British Association for Counselling
37a Sheep Street
Rugby
Warks CV21 3BY
Tel 01788 578328

British Association of Nutritional Therapists
PO Box 47
Heathfield
East Sussex TN21 8ZX

British Holistic Medical Association
179 Gloucester Place
London NW1 6DX
Tel 0171 262 5299

British Massage Therapy Council
Greenbank House
65a Adelphi Street
Preston
Lancs PR1 7BH
Tel 01772 881063

British Wheel of Yoga
1 Hamilton Place
Boston Road
Sleaford
Lincs NG34 7ES
Tel 01529 306851

Candida Support Network
Gibliston Mill
Colinsburgh
Leven
Fife
Scotland KY9 1JS
Tel 0133 340311
A UK database has been set up to put fellow sufferers living near each other in touch, in order for them to meet up informally, or to set up a support group. Details of up and running groups are also given. Send £5 and a sae to the above address.

Candida Workshops UK
For locations and dates contact:
Gibliston Mill
Colinsburgh
Leven
Fife
Scotland KY9 1JS

Tel 01333 340311 or 0171 428 9577
One-day workshops to give the practical know-how and holistic understanding that will help in treating candida problems.

Candida Web Site
http://ourworld.compuserve.com/homepages/candida
For workshop details, support group contacts, details of books and tapes, treatments and research.

Council for Complementary and Alternative Medicine
179 Gloucester Place
London NW1 6DX
Tel 0171 237 5165
Fax 0171 237 5175

Diagnostech
The Cottage
Lakeside
180 Lifford Lane
Kings Norton
B30 3NT
Tel 0121 458 3407
Fax 0121 459 1656
For testing: Yeast Screen-CandaScan, CS1 Stool Culture for Yeast and Mucosal Barrier Screen.

General Council and Register of Naturopaths
2 Goswell Road
Street
Somerset BA16 OJG
Tel 01458 840072

Institute for Complementary Medicine and British Register of Complementary Practitioners
PO Box 194
London SE16 1QZ
Tel 0171 237 5165
Fax 0171 237 5175

National Institute of Medical Herbalists
56 Longbrook Street
Exeter
Devon EX4 6AH
Tel 01392 426022
Fax 01392 498963

NLP – International Teaching Seminars
Ian McDermott
Director of Training
7 Rudall Crescent
London NW3 1RS
Tel 0181 442 4133
Fax 0181 442 4155
Ian McDermott is training a core of NLP practitioners who will specialize in health issues.

Register of Nutritional Therapists Ltd
Hatton Green
Warwick CV35 7LA

Society of Homoeopaths
2 Artisan Road
Northampton NN1 4HU
Tel 01604 21400

Specialist Practitioners
A directory of complementary practitioners who treat Candida albicans holistically is incorporated in Jane McWhirter's excellent book The Practical Guide to Candida, *published by All Hallows House Foundation.*

The Terrence Higgins Trust
52–54 Grays Inn Road
London WC1X 8JU
Tel 0171 831 0330
Helpline 0171 242 1010

For help with and information about HIV and AIDS related issues.

UK Homoeopathic Medical Association
6 Livingstone Road
Gravesend
Kent DA12 5DZ
Tel 01474 560336

Yoga Biomedical Trust
Yoga Therapy Centre
3rd Floor
Royal London Homoeopathic Hospital Trust
60 Great Ormond Street
London WC1N 3HR
Tel 0171 833 7267
Fax 0171 833 7292.

Useful further reading

BOOKS ON CANDIDA

Beat Candida Through Diet, Gill Jacobs and Joanna Kjaer (Vermillion, 1997).

Candida albicans, Leon Chaitow, ND, DO (Thorsons, 1996).

Chronic Candidiasis – The Yeast Syndrome, Michael T. Murray, ND (Prima, 1997).

Overcoming Candida: The Ultimate Cookery Guide, Xandria Williams (Element Books, 1998)

The Practical Guide to Candida and UK directory, Jane McWhirter (All Hallows House Foundation, 1995).

The Yeast Connection, William G. Crook, MD (Professional Books Inc and Vintage Books, 1996).

The Yeast Connection and the Woman, William G. Crook, MD (Professional Books Inc, 1997).

For plenty of sound advice on what you can eat on an anti-candida diet, the following are particularly recommended: *Beat Candida Through Diet*, *Diet to Help Candida*, *Overcoming Candida: The Ultimate Cookery Guide* and *The Practical Guide to Candida*

GENERAL READING

Autogenic Training, Dr Kai Kermani (Souvenir Press, 1990).

Beat Fatigue with Yoga, Fiona Agombar (Element,1999).

Consumer Guide to Vitamins, Angela Dowden and Graham Lacey (Pan Books, 1996).

Dr Braly's Optimum Health Program, James Braly, MD (Times Books, 1995).

Eat Right 4 Your Type, Peter D'Adamo, MD (Putnam, 1996).

Enter the Zone, Barry Sears, PhD, with Bill Lawren (Regan, 1995)

Food Combining for Health, Doris Grant and Jean Joice (Thorsons, 1984).

Glutamine, The Ultimate Nutrient, Judy Shabert, MD, RD. and Nancy Ehrlich (Avery, 1994).

The Healing Power of Illness, Thorwald Dethlefsen and Dr Rudiger Dahlke, MD (Element, 1995).

NLP and Health, Ian McDermott and Joseph O'Connor (Thorsons, 1996).

Nutritional Health Bible, Linda Lazarides (Thorsons, 1997).

Principles of Yoga, Cheryl Isaacson (Thorsons, 1996).

Probiotics, Leon Chaitow, ND, and Natasha Trenev (Thorsons, 1990).

The Rotation Diet Cookbook, Jill Carter and Alison Edwards (Element Books, 1997)

Total Wellness, Joseph Pizzorno, ND (Prima,1996).

Vibrational Medicine, Richard Gerber, MD (Bear and Company, 1988).

You can Heal Your Life, Louise Hay (Eden Grove, 1996).

For HIV and AIDS-related issues: *Continuum* magazine, 172 Foundling Court, Brunswick Centre, London WC1N 1QE, Tel 0171 713 7071.

Index